MW00626130

On Being a Veterinarian

Book 1:

What to Expect, How to Prepare

April Kung, DVM

Content disclaimer: Any incidents recounted in this series that are based on true occurrences have had select details altered to protect confidentiality. Suggestions made are based on the author's personal experience and research. Author claims no professional training or education in psychiatry, psychology, human nutrition, exercise physiology, or medical education. Please consult a certified or licensed expert in these areas for professional help. Any advice on veterinary medical practice provided by the author is intended for application by licensed veterinarians capable of using their own medical judgment. Do not attempt to use any medical advice provided by the author without a medical degree. In no event should the author be responsible or liable, directly or indirectly, for any damage or loss caused or alleged to be caused by, or in connection with, the use of or reliance on any such information provided by the author. Health-related topics, legal and financial information provided by the author should not be substituted for professional medical, legal and financial advice. It is your responsibility to research the accuracy, completeness and usefulness of all opinions and other information provided by the author. The author assumes no responsibility or liability for any consequence resulting, directly or indirectly, for any action or inaction taken based on or made in reliance on the information provided.

Published by Happy Animal Productions
First Edition December 2017
ISBN-13: 978-1-948356-00-8

Table of Contents

Acknowledgements

I am forever indebted to my dear friend and colleague, **Kerry Kraemer, DVM,** and to my dear friend, former client and retired cardiac nurse, **Denise Urquijo**, for reading every laborious draft without complaint, and for cheerily encouraging me to continue when I felt so discouraged I wanted to quit. Many thanks also to the pre-veterinary and veterinary students, and other veterinarians whose feedback helped shape this work. I am blessed to have in my life my psychiatrist, **Harold Figueroa, MD**, because he taught me to like myself and to love my life, which made the pursuit of this endeavor possible. I am deeply grateful to my mentor and cherished friend, **Alicia Ragni, DVM,** for her faith in me, when I had none, and for going through my writing line by line, improving both the style and substance of the books in this series. To my sister, **Eva Lawrence, Ph.D.**, I owe a huge debt of gratitude for the inspiration she has always been to me, for her insightful and incisive editorial assistance, which has made me a better writer, and for the countless hours she spent sourcing academic articles and helping me to better understand and explain psychology concepts that were out of my league. Finally, I would like to thank my husband, **Alex Jacobs, MD**, for believing in me, and for his love and essential guidance throughout this project. He pushed me to think more deeply about what I was *really* trying to say. Sometimes, at personal cost to himself due to my irritation with him, he prevented me from believing I'd already said what I'd really wanted to say - when I hadn't. His support gave me the space I needed to wrestle demons and wring ideas out of air, and he asked only a few home cooked meals in return. I lament I haven't time to say more nice things about him, but I have to get started on dinner...

Dedication

*"He is your friend, your partner, your defender, your dog.
You are his life, his love, his leader. He will be yours,
faithful and true, to the last beat of his heart. You owe it
to him to be worthy of such devotion."*

- Unknown

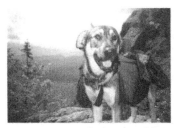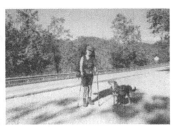

**In Loving Memory of Monte
(September 1997 – June 8, 2012)**

In the spring of 1998, before the dream of becoming a veterinarian had entered my mind, I set out to hike the Appalachian Trail with Monte. He was nine months old. We started at the northern terminus of The Hundred Mile Wilderness in Maine, and hiked south.

Monte carried his backpack and his bedroll, and I carried mine. I had never hiked before. Not like this. Not with a heavy backpack that contained everything I needed to survive in the woods for weeks.

Monte didn't enjoy carrying the heavy weight of his pack any more than I enjoyed carrying mine. For the first week, every morning when I packed up our gear and called him to me so I could put his pack on, he would run away, or he would roll over. It was a daily battle of wills.

About halfway through The Hundred Mile Wilderness, as we were struggling up and down a series of four mountains, White Cap, Hay, West Peak, and Gulf Hagas, we encountered an almost impassable obstacle. At the top of Hay Mountain was a blowdown of what must have been a hundred pine trees. A violent storm had hit that peak the previous winter. Since most hikers hoping to hike the entire 2,200 miles of the A.T. begin in the south, in Georgia, trail maintenance crews hadn't yet cleared this section of the trail.

I had had the terrifying experience several days prior of losing the trail completely after trying to bypass a much less impressive blowdown. That day, I'd searched vainly for the trail for over an hour before finally resigning myself to starving to death in the wilderness. I sat down in the dry, brown leaves that covered the forest floor, and cried. I called to Monte who was sitting with his back to me about 300 yards away. He wouldn't come. Finally, I went to him and discovered why he wouldn't heed my call. He had found the trail.

The trail, I learned, was like a lifeline, winding its way through a 65,000-acre forest that looked the same in every direction. It would disorient you at the first opportunity, and was indifferent to human tears. I would not risk losing the trail again. We wouldn't go around this blowdown. We were just going to have to go through it.

At first, we tried doing it with our packs on, but Monte and I both kept getting caught on branches, and we often couldn't squeeze between the skeletal remains of the trees at all. So I took my pack off, then I took Monte's off. He was elated to be free of his heavy burden, and he zipped through the maze of trunks, branches and pine needles like a happy little mouse. I had to push and pull both of our packs through the wreckage, climbing over and under the trunks and branches, inch by miserable inch.

When I emerged on the other side almost an hour later, I was covered with sweat and blood. I'd received hundreds of scratches from the sharp twigs and prickly needles, and the sweat seeping into the wounds stung me all over my face and arms. I put on my pack, trying to make a strong showing, but when I lifted Monte's pack and called for him, he ran away, as he always did.

I started wailing and crying like a big baby. I wanted to die. I wanted lightning to strike me, to vaporize me. I was exhausted. I was hungry. I was scared, and we were on our own in the middle of a hundred miles of wilderness.

When Monte saw me standing there, holding his pack and crying, he stopped and stared at me. He cocked his head for a moment as if thinking very hard. Then he walked back to me and sat down right in front of me as if to say, "It's okay. You put that pack on me now. I'll carry it." And he let me put it on him without anymore struggle.

In fact, after that day, he never resisted having his pack put on again. Months later, soon after returning to our lives in the world of soft beds and plentiful food, a veterinarian diagnosed Monte with a traumatically luxated knee cap. Despite the pain he must have been in, he carried that backpack hundreds of miles, up and down mountains, because he knew I needed him to.

He was the best friend I ever had. He was my soul mate from the moment I carried him as a puppy, terrified and trembling, out of the shelter, to the moment, fourteen years later, when I held him in my arms and said goodbye forever as he died. I miss him every day, and will continue to miss him to the end of my days.

My deepest hope is that this series will inspire and empower future veterinary doctors to continue doing the essential but difficult work of practicing veterinary medicine - with boundless compassion for their patients and for themselves - for the sake of other inherently worthy animals, like Monte, who love without limit, and live at our mercy.

On Being a Veterinarian: Series Introduction

Dear Future Colleague;

If you want to be a veterinarian you're in good company. People who want to be veterinarians tend to be, on the whole, kind hearted and empathetic. The world needs more people like you.

If you have what it takes to actually become a veterinarian (the grades, the wit, the grit) then you're in an even more elite group. Congratulations! You're the crème de la crème! You're probably one of those rare, lucky people who can do whatever you want with your life, and if becoming a vet is what you're setting your mind to, I've little doubt you'll succeed.

I'm proud to be a Doctor of Veterinary Medicine (DVM) and I feel sincerely fortunate and honored to be a part of a community of professionals that consistently forms statistical clusters at the right end of the bell curve on all kinds of great characteristics, such as intelligence, integrity, conscientiousness, dedication, and compassion.

Additionally, medicine is an exceptional field of knowledge and the very process of attaining that specialized knowledge has reshaped my neural pathways for the better. It has enabled me to understand the world more objectively, to think more rationally and to see things more clearly. My mother once told me that she didn't know how to think until after she took calculus. That's how I feel about medicine.

Furthermore, being a veterinarian is just plain cool. Most people think veterinarians are the cat's pajamas. My husband is an MD, and when people we meet find out what he does, the reaction is positive but reserved - a thoughtful, "huh" accompanied by a respectful nod.

When people find out what I do, their whole posture changes. It's as if an electrical current suddenly surged from their feet up to their head. They stand up straighter, quiver a little, and I get the feeling they're desperately trying not to hug me. They lean in, open their eyes wide and say something like, "Oh, wow! I always wanted to be a veterinarian!" Then they proceed to tell me all about their beloved pets.

Here's another neat thing about being a veterinarian: If Armageddon hits, we should all be so lucky as to have a medical doctor around, and the best kind of doctor to have on your post-apocalypse team is a veterinarian. Why? Because, unlike medical doctors who treat only humans, and who specialize on a narrow subset within the wider field of medicine, such as ophthalmology or radiology, most veterinary doctors have to maintain competence in all medical subjects from cardiology and nephrology to gastroenterology and ophthalmology to surgery.

When I was in the movie theater watching *Avatar,* and Sigourney Weaver's character was dying from a gunshot wound to the abdomen, I knew that the bullet had perforated her intestinal tract and she needed emergency surgery to survive. Of all the kinds of MDs in the world, only an MD surgeon could have saved her. "But," I marveled to myself, "I could have saved her." And you know what? That's an amazing feeling.

However, this isn't going to be a James Herriot or Dr. Doolittle-like series filled with heartwarming stories of colorful characters and animal filled adventures intended mainly to entertain. Instead, this series of books is a no holds barred, down and dirty, tell it like it is, factual account of the intellectual, emotional and psychological realities of being a small animal veterinarian. It's a series of candid, personal letters from me, an experienced veterinarian who has worked as an emergency vet, a general practice vet and a relief vet, to you – the future small animal veterinarian.

These books are meant for anyone who is anything like the person I used to be. That is, you want to be a veterinarian because you care about and want to help animals. You have a relentless driving desire to understand the science and art of medicine. And you're so excited about the prospect of one day wearing that white coat and being called "doctor" as you step up to save your first patient, that no one and nothing can deter you from your goal.

You are a sledgehammer, a bullet train, a jet engine, and an 800-pound gorilla rolled into one. You have Superman's laser vision enabling you, forsaking all else, to focus intensely on and burn through anything between you and your goal. If this is you, fantastic - because that's what it's going to take. But that's not all it's going to take.

The road you've chosen is a hard one, not merely because of the intellectual challenges of mastering organic chemistry or physiology, and not merely because of the logistical challenges of completing the multitudinous administrative requirements just to apply to veterinary school. Yes, these things are hard, but for an apt candidate, in all honesty, they require little more than dedicated focus, good organizational skills and some common sense. The truth is - the biggest hurdles on the road you've chosen are the emotional and psychological challenges you will face during and after veterinary school - and these are what I want to prepare you for.

There is an amazing sense of kinship between veterinarians. We feel a bond with each other that bridges generational, geographical and cultural barriers. It's a feeling of empathy and warmth that springs from intuiting the essential goodness in another person, and from knowing we share the same desire to serve animals and society from a place of profound compassion and integrity.

The fact that you're reading this book tells me you're of the same ilk, and I feel the same protective instinct, the same desire to help and support you, as I do for my veterinarian colleagues.

Since graduating from veterinary school, I have experienced many surprises. I've encountered countless situations and confronted dozens of revelations for which I had not been prepared. Advanced knowledge could have improved this journey for me. Since I can think of no good reason why this knowledge shouldn't be available to others embarking on this journey, my mission is to provide it. I recently became a member of a Facebook group for veterinarians. Reading the posts of other veterinarians in this group strengthened my conviction that what I want to say to aspiring veterinarians desperately needs to be said.

Putting in my hours as a veterinary assistant to qualify for vet school, I helped restrain patients, cleaned cages, walked dogs, took out the trash, vacuumed, and mopped. In return, I got to observe all the goings-on behind the scenes at several veterinary hospitals. As a part of my application to vet school, I wrote this in my personal essay:

"I must continually suppress the urge to barrage the veterinarians with whom I work with the hundreds of questions that are constantly running through my mind. Was toxicity a suspicion when this animal first presented? If you had treated on that assumption, might the animal have survived or was the metabolism of the toxin too far advanced to remedy? Does this radiograph indicate that the bullet shattered upon entry? What symptoms indicate to you that internal hemorrhaging is a possibility? Why is it not a given despite the hematuria?

Is it possible that ultrasound won't be revealing? Is exploratory surgery an option?"

In retrospect, I'd say these were pretty good questions, but I wouldn't have gained much had I actually asked them. The medical education required to answer these questions myself would come soon enough, and without the medical education, any answers provided would have been lost on me. I realize now those questions stemmed from an intense and frustrated craving to know exactly what was really going on inside the heads of the doctors as they worked beside me. So anemic was my understanding of what it meant to be a doctor though, that I was incapable of even imagining the questions I should have asked.

From my perspective today, I can see very clearly the nature of the divide between me, the veterinary assistant, and the veterinarians. Even though I worked with them, assisted them and talked with them, even though I watched as they performed surgery or an emergency cut-down procedure to get an IV line in a critical patient, so vast was the chasm between what I thought it meant to be a veterinarian and what I know now that I may as well have been in a different dimension or a different universe. That gap of understanding could only have been bridged had I been able to read their minds.

My craving to know the hidden, inner world of veterinary doctors led me to read many books written by DVMs, as well as MDs. These books never failed to fascinate, but they were written mainly to entertain a mass audience. The truly great and ambitious ones, such as Atul Gawande's *Complications*, sought to educate as well as entertain, but, still being written for a mass audience, even the exceptional books didn't speak in practical terms to future doctors, and certainly, they offered no practical advice to future veterinarians.

When I began working on this project, my initial intention was to write a single book for the express benefit of aspiring veterinarians that would cover every aspect of what it's like to be a veterinarian from my perspective as a small animal DVM. However, halfway through the first draft of the first chapter, it became clear there was simply too much to say. I didn't want to provide merely a generalized overview that seemed helpful on the surface but left you without concrete understanding or actionable knowledge. I wanted to give you a comprehensive precognizance – the opportunity to read my mind, so to speak – so you could navigate the same road I traveled, but with greater success and less stress.

If I attempted to include all of this information in a single book, it would overwhelm rather than educate and inform. Therefore, I decided to write a series of mini-books, each providing an in-depth view into a separate topic relevant to future small animal veterinarians. The underlying objective of every book in the *On Being a Veterinarian* series is to increase your chances of feeling happy and fulfilled in your future career by giving you a glimpse of that future now.

Because of the in-depth nature and practical intent of the information I provide, this book series is likely to be most helpful to pre-veterinary tracking undergraduate students, veterinary students or new veterinary graduates with an interest in small animal medicine. I practice in the United States, so if you live in a different country, some of the advice I offer, or experiences I recount, may not be applicable where you live. While I'd be happy if experienced veterinarians enjoy this series, or if people in the general public who are merely curious find something of interest in these pages, these are not my primary objectives.

If it's true that hindsight is 20/20, and I believe it is, then my purpose is to repackage my own hindsight as a veterinarian and offer it to you, future doctor, in the form of foresight. I want you to be prepared in advance for the challenges ahead, rather than surprised and taken off guard. I want to help you face these challenges with grace and equanimity.

I got my driver's license over thirty years ago – long before GPS technology was available to the public. Depending on your age, you may never have had the unnerving experience of driving to an unfamiliar destination without knowing for sure if you were on the right road, or even if you were going in the right direction. Not only was there no GPS, at that time, only the rich and famous had cellular phones. I can tell you, it could be very stressful, regardless of whether you were trying to find your way in a bustling big city, or out in the sticks where the empty roads were not only nameless but also seemingly endless.

Driving in unfamiliar territory always made me feel anxious and vulnerable. My mind would race with thoughts like, 'Did I miss the turn? I've had my eyes peeled this whole time, so I don't know how I could have missed it, but it feels like I've been on this road for way too long. Should I stop at the next gas station to ask directions? What kind of neighborhood is this? Is it safe?'

If I was lucky enough to get directions from a helpful gas station attendant, the best directions always included references to prominent landmarks. Once I spotted one of those landmarks, all the rigidity and tension would leave my body. My stress level would drop as if a heavy stone had been pushed off my chest. I'd take a deep breath, exhale with relief and think, 'Oh thank goodness! I'm going the right way! Everything is okay!' Like those gas station attendants did for me, if I can reduce the level of stress you experience by telling you about the notable landmarks you'll encounter on your journey, I will consider my time writing these books well spent.

This series will combine narrative, both fiction and non-fiction, with instructive sections such as those you may expect to find in self-help books. I've chosen this hybrid structure to provide explanation coupled with (I hope) some entertainment, as well as specific resources and tools to help make your journey an adventure to enjoy rather than a hardship to endure. If you have your heart set on becoming a veterinarian, I want you to be the best, the most fulfilled and happiest veterinarian you can possibly be – both for your sake and for the sake of the animals who will depend on you.

In a June 2015 Veterinary Economics article, Dr. Dean Scott, a practicing veterinarian for 35 years, said,

"When people enter the veterinary field, we are flat out not prepared for the mental stress that the job entails... When I was a teenager, some veterinarians gave soft warnings about the job, but what I have encountered was so much more than they hinted at."

Dr. Scott's lament is far from uncommon. This is why I've decided to reveal the hidden realities of what being a small animal veterinarian is actually like. In order to thrive as a veterinarian, you're going to need more than a hint. You need someone to pull back the curtain and prepare you for the side of veterinary medicine that only veterinarians know about.

My intent is to be as candid as possible. This means I may reveal things about my experiences that are uncomfortable to talk about. Sometimes what I write may cast others in an unflattering light, sometimes I will tell you things that make me look bad. I have no intention of causing harm or insulting anyone, nor do I seek to make myself look better than I actually am. I'm human, you're human, anyone who could possibly read this book is human. We are imperfect creatures in an imperfect world doing the best we can with what we have at any given moment.

My single motivating purpose for any disclosure is to help you avoid mistakes I've made, or that I've seen others make, or to prepare you to confront unavoidable difficulties in proactive and positive ways. Underlying that motivation, aside from my fondness for science and animal loving nerds (or geeks, if you prefer), is my desire to see the field of veterinary medicine filled with happy, self-respecting, emotionally resilient, and successful practitioners who are driven and empowered to provide the level of care and compassion every animal deserves.

I think the single, most important insight you should take away after reading the books in this series is that realizing the dream of becoming a veterinarian is only half the battle. Mastering the reality of that dream after you achieve it is the other half, and that requires a clear view of the road ahead; a view unclouded by misperceptions and faulty expectations.

I'm no spring chicken, and veterinary medicine is not my first rodeo. Before college, I waited tables, managed a cookie shop, was an aerobics instructor, and even tried my hand at selling vacuum cleaners door-to-door, among other things. After my first college degree, I worked in corporate advertising, point of sale promotions, internal corporate communications, historic real estate rehabilitation, and started, ran and sold my own pet-sitting business. I've had the opportunity to travel and live abroad and to learn about many different cultures, and before veterinary school, I hiked hundreds of miles on the Appalachian Trail with Monte. Throughout this series, I will draw on, not only my experience as a veterinarian, but all of my personal and professional experiences to give you the best of what I've learned as it pertains to your aspirations.

Fair warning: I use terms or refer to scientific concepts you may not yet have encountered in your studies. Lack of familiarity with these things will not prevent you from benefitting from these books, though I hope I may inspire you to investigate any concepts you're not yet familiar with. My writing also includes quite a few sci-fi allusions. If you're not familiar with these references, please indulge this science and animal loving nerd.

I'll be releasing each new book as it's finished. I haven't given myself a set schedule, because the topics are numerous and complex, and I would prefer to have sufficient time to explore and present them adequately, rather than feeling I have to meet a deadline. If you want to be informed as each new book in the series is published, please go to my website www.realize.vet and subscribe to my email list.

This series introduction is also available for free on my website. Feel free to download and share it with anyone.

Kindest regards,
Dr. K
Flagstaff, Arizona

On Being a Veterinarian: Book 1 Preface

This book exposes the chasm between what people think it will be like to be a veterinarian and the reality of what it's actually like to be a veterinarian, so future veterinary doctors can better prepare for the realities of this very challenging, but potentially very fulfilling, career. Some have taken to referring to veterinary medicine as a "calling," rather than a career, because a calling is something you were born to do and must do.

However, inherent in the idea that veterinary medicine is a calling is the very dangerous belief that those of us called to be veterinarians must be willing to make any and every sacrifice for our calling. It begins with the intense rigors of undergraduate science courses, and then continues through veterinary school and into medical practice.

We sacrifice time with our friends and family. We sacrifice hobbies and all the sunny, inspiring dreams we once had about the amazing future we envisioned. We sacrifice time to care for ourselves. We sacrifice to work

harder, work longer, give more, try harder, be better...
But still, we're not good enough. Still, we don't live up to
this calling.

I wrote this book to disabuse you of the illusion that
it's possible to live up to this calling. Veterinary medicine
is not perfect, and therefore no one can ever hope to be
a perfect veterinarian. The road to clinical competence is
longer and harder than you think. It's also endless. So, I
want you to throw away the idea that if you just sacrifice
enough, someday, you'll live up to the ideal. You can't.
No one can.

You also shouldn't live *for* this calling. If you try,
it will take everything you have and still demand
more. Medicine is a jealous mistress. If you don't set
boundaries, she will consume you. Your greatest
accomplishment as a future veterinary doctor will be in
learning how to live *with* this calling. And the only way to
live *with* this calling is to pace yourself, be patient with
yourself, be kind to yourself, and take care of yourself.

What You Might Expect

"In theory there is no difference between theory and practice. In practice there is."
-Yogi Berra

Imagine this: You've already made it through four strenuous, sleep deprived years of veterinary school. You've passed the National and State Boards despite the trembling anxiety you felt the day of those tests. You've jumped through myriad paperwork hoops to attain your state and DEA licenses, and most importantly, after several interviews where you grew progressively more practiced at appearing confident and ready, you successfully secured your first job!

Today is your first day as a real doctor. Just to have made it this far, truly, you are a superhero. You should be incredibly proud of what you've accomplished. You are now a member of an extremely elite and well educated group who comprise only about 0.03% of the world's population:[21] Veterinary Medical Doctors.

Despite feeling some trepidation, which is only normal, there is a little voice in your head assuring you that everything you learned in veterinary school has prepared you to practice medicine. In fact, this little voice, which may sound just like one of your favorite vet school professors, will tell you that since you are newly graduated, you have the distinct advantage of possessing the most up to date medical knowledge available.

On my first day as a new veterinarian, this little voice was the only thing that kept me from collapsing into a sobbing ball of cowardice and rolling home. So, definitely indulge that little voice because it will give you the courage you need. But I want you to be prepared for this reality, too: If you thought veterinary school was hard, you ain't seen nothin' yet.

Applying what we learned in veterinary school to real medical cases in the real world is very difficult for a new veterinarian. I know you don't expect it to be easy. If you wanted an easy job you wouldn't be thinking of becoming a veterinarian. But perhaps I can make it little easier by preparing you for the nature of the challenge.

As a new veterinarian, I felt very frustrated with myself because, even though I had all this knowledge in my head, I was unable to use it in the graceful way I intended. In the novel *Madame Bovary*, Gustave Flaubert writes, "Human speech is like a cracked kettle on which we tap crude rhythms for bears to dance to, while we long to make music that will melt the stars."

The nature of my frustration stemmed from a similar, unfulfilled longing. I struggled for a long time trying to figure out why it was so hard for me to apply the elegant, logical medical knowledge in my brain in a way that would do it justice. I think I've finally come up with an apt analogy.

Have you ever had to move? Why do you think moving is said to be one of the most stressful experiences in life? I think it's because we have to pack everything we own, everything that is precious to us, and all the things we use on a daily basis, into boxes and bags and suitcases.

Whether we're moving cross country or just to a different place in the same neighborhood, once we arrive, we have to unpack all those things and put them in new places in our new home. The more possessions we have, the longer this process takes and the greater the duration of our discomfort as we attempt to live our day-to-day lives with some semblance of normalcy despite the fact we can't find our underwear.

Moving from veterinary school to your first job as a veterinarian is like this. Imagine the sum total of every physical object in a large, five bedroom, three and a half bathroom house is the symbolic equivalent of the sum total of every single thing you'll learn in four years of veterinary school. Each household object represents one piece of knowledge. There are some heavy, foundational pieces of knowledge, like acid-base equilibrium. Big concepts like this can be likened to refrigerators, laundry machines or large sectional couches. There are also many little things like the histopathological appearance of cryptosporidium in the small intestine. These kinds of factoids can be likened to paperclips or random pennies from under the couch. Then there's everything in between: Clothes, bookshelves, computers, lamps, bath mats, the dining room table, extension cords, boxes of random hardware you never knew what to do with, and still don't, but can't bring yourself to throw away. You get the picture.

Now, imagine that every time you learn something in vet school, it's like taking one of those household objects and packing it into a giant moving truck. After all, you know veterinary school is only temporary, and when it's over you're going to move on to a new life in a new place. Sometimes what you pack in this giant truck is a big heavy object, and sometimes it's not, but you do your best to make efficient use of the space because you know it all has to fit in this one truck.

As the classes, semesters and years tick by, this giant moving truck gradually gets filled to capacity with all manner of essential medical knowledge, as well as some stuff you're not sure will ever be useful but you're packing it anyway - just in case. When the big day finally comes, and vet school is over, your giant moving truck is crammed full. After you pull down the roll up door at the back of the truck, and secure it with a padlock, you climb into the driver's seat and motor on to your new home.

When you first begin practicing, it's going to feel very similar to how it feels when you move to a new place but haven't finished unpacking yet. Everything you need, all of your veterinary knowledge is inside that giant truck, you just won't be sure exactly *where*. You might see a sick cat with chronic kidney disease and hyperthyroidism and think, 'Well now, I know I packed kidney disease in the same box as urology, but where did I put that box of hyperthyroidism? I could have sworn it was right next to the box of diabetes. And why, oh why, didn't I pack fluid therapy in the same box as kidney disease? Where on Earth did I put fluid therapy anyway? Is it in the box labeled "septic shock?" Or maybe it's in the box labeled "CPR."' Just as you locate the information on fluid therapy - but before you've had a chance to unpack it - a dog will come in with a history of eating rat poison and you'll be racking your brain to remember where in that giant truck you put your box of toxicology.

On top of this, everything you learned in veterinary school will be stored in separate, discreet folders that correspond with the classes you took, such as "Pathology," "Cardiology" or "Gastroenterology." Your patients will not present according to these neat and discrete categories but your brain will consistently attempt to treat them as if they have. The rigid structure of your academic knowledge base will be so ingrained that in many cases you will not even be aware of your mental mistakes until later. Until you amass sufficient real-world experience to bridge the artificial separations between medical subjects, your brain will superimpose that fictitious mental scaffold onto every case you encounter.

Grasping a concept in veterinary school is very different from being able to apply that concept in the real world. In veterinary school, you will remember information in the way that best enables you to correctly answer exam questions. It will take time for you to unpack everything you learned and rearrange it in a way that is useful to you as a practicing clinician. When you begin your career as a veterinarian and experience these frustrations, I want you to remember that this is all normal. There is nothing wrong with you. Be patient with yourself.

What You Don't Expect

"Life is so constructed, that the event does not, cannot, will not, match the expectation."
\- Charlotte Bronte

While you may expect the difficulties you'll face as you try to apply what you learned in vet school to real medical cases in the real world, what most new vets don't see coming are the emotional and psychological difficulties of being a new doctor. Yes, you were granted the degree of Doctor of Veterinary Medicine. Yes, you were hired as a doctor. Yes, everyone calls you doctor. But you don't feel like a doctor. And yet, suddenly, you have all of the responsibilities of this role. It's this aspect of becoming a veterinarian that I most want to prepare you for, and what the bulk of this book is truly about.

The term for the emotional and psychological reaction you will experience when you first begin practicing is transition shock. Transition shock is a known phenomenon in many industries, especially the health care industry. The term is most commonly used in reference to the stress and moral distress that result from changes in professional, social, intellectual, and developmental roles as graduating nurses move from an academic to a professional environment.[1] The term has also been applied, though less frequently, to what human doctors experience as they transition from the role of student to practicing doctor.[18] The reason transition shock happens less often in doctors practicing human medicine is discussed briefly later. I've never actually heard the term used in veterinary medicine, but taking into consideration my own experience, the many personal conversations I've had with other veterinarians and the reading I've done on this topic, I will take the liberty here of asserting that transition shock is absolutely what occurs when newly graduated veterinarians begin to practice.

Probably the most common phrase I hear from new veterinarians - and the phrase I remember saying myself - is: "I had no idea what I was getting myself into." That's the *shock* of transition shock, and it's the treacherous part of the problem. It's the teeth of the monster. I aim to defang this beast for you. I want to eliminate the shock so that when the time comes, you will experience merely a transition (albeit a difficult one), but with no surprises and no disillusionment. And when your time comes to make this transition, you will know that what you're feeling is what we all feel when we first start out, and you are not alone.

A dry, academic treatise on the causes, signs and sequelae of this insidious pathology, however, will not adequately protect you. It would enter your cerebral cortex, your thinking brain, and then it would merely sit there politely amidst thoughts of Avogadro's Number, the Linnaean Classification System and every other dispassionate memory gleaned from your prerequisite science classes. We need to build your resistance in the part of your brain that transition shock actually affects; not the cerebral cortex but the limbic system, the emotional brain.

We're going to use the basic principles of vaccinology to inoculate you: By exposing you to a low dose simulation of the causes of transition shock, we will be preparing your emotional immune system to recognize later exposure. This is called "stress inoculation."[6] It's a technique used in clinical psychotherapy.

This stress inoculation is going to be delivered in the form of a story about you in the future. To boost the effectiveness of this prophylaxis, you should do your best to participate in this story by using creative visualization. Picture yourself inside this story as if it's happening right now. Let your imagination add colors, sounds, scents, and any other details that make the story feel more real to you. Make every attempt to acknowledge, accept and fully experience every physical sensation and every emotion this story inspires in you.

Your First Day as a Doctor

You have just graduated from veterinary school. After walking across a brightly lit stage to the sound of well earned applause and being handed your Doctor of Veterinary Medicine degree by the smiling Dean of your college, you become acutely aware of a huge weight lifted from your shoulders. All of the long days in lecture, the long nights afterwards of intense study, the struggle to stay awake in class despite chronic sleep deprivation, the stress of exam after exam after exam, the 16+ hour workdays and constant pressure of clinical rotations... Four of the hardest years of your life... Poof! Over. Done.

In the green summer gardens outside the amphitheater, there are hugs and handshakes with professors and school administrators who encouraged you, and photographs and tear-filled goodbyes with classmates who have been your study partners, close friends and support system throughout this arduous journey. Now you must each go your separate ways, find your own paths, and forge ahead alone in your new careers.

Despite the bittersweet end of this intense chapter of your life, you're eager to move ahead, and full of optimism and confidence. Nothing you ever encounter again in your life will be as challenging as veterinary school - and you climbed that mountain like it was Mount Doom and you were carrying the One Ring of Sauron.

You start the job search in earnest. You're fortunate to be offered a position right away. Your family is so proud of you. You post the great news on Facebook. The practice owner where you're going to work has been a vet for thirty years! He promised to mentor you so you won't have to worry about getting in over your head, or having to figure everything out for yourself right away. Just thinking about how much you're going to learn from him is elating. Your new life as a doctor has begun. You feel like you've swallowed a whole year of sunshine.

You spend your first week in the hospital shadowing your boss and the two other doctors who work there, following them around, observing how they interact with clients and support staff. You experience an almost guilty thrill every time someone introduces you as "Doctor." You make small talk with new colleagues to begin breaking the ice. You play around a little with the medical record software system. The head technician gives you a rundown of the in-house laboratory equipment. The Practice Manager puts your name in the computer system. The receptionist spends some time going over the phone system with you. You fill out tax withholding and automatic deposit forms.

The following week you finally get to be "The Doctor." You're nervous but elated to begin applying all of those amazing things you learned about in veterinary school. You've arrived to the hospital early, and now as you watch the clock tick down to 8AM, when the first patients will be placed in exam rooms to wait for you, you feel like a race horse waiting for the gates to open.

You've looked over your schedule. You have nine appointments today, one hour for each appointment. They're going easy on you this week, except that all your appointments are sick visits. You know that can't be helped. Wellness and vaccine visits were scheduled way in advance with your boss.

The first four appointments are a middle-aged male cat that is urinating in inappropriate places in the house, a geriatric dog that is limping, a young bulldog who has been incessantly shaking her head, and a coughing Chihuahua. By the time you've seen your fourth patient it is evident your boss doesn't have time to help you with your cases. You have so many questions, each case seems to generate at least twenty of them, but you have to limit your questions to just the most critical, because you can only ask during the course of the few minutes you catch him leaving one exam room before entering the next.

You end up having to make most of the decisions completely on your own. Is it okay to prescribe this medication even though the client refuses to let you run any diagnostics? The liver enzymes of this patient are elevated but how elevated do they need to be before you should worry about prescribing a medication for his arthritis? Should you send home ear medications for this dog even though no one could hold her still and you weren't able get the otoscope in her ear to make sure her eardrum was intact? Could you be misinterpreting the radiograph on this coughing Chihuahua? Maybe it's heart failure and not pneumonia? Will pneumonia always present with a fever and an elevated white blood cell count?

Meanwhile, despite the longer appointments, you're still falling behind schedule because it's taking you so long to work through every case. You know you're spending too much time talking to your clients, but they all just seem to want to keep talking and talking. It's been hard for you to get them to answer your questions.

"Is any urine coming out when Fluffy tries to pee or is he just straining and straining? Is he still eating? Is he still acting normal?"

The owners argue with each other over the answers. Mr. says, "Yes, I saw urine in the litter box." Mrs. says, "No, that was from the other cat." Then they want to tell you all sorts of things that have nothing to do with why Fluffy came in today, or even about Fluffy at all. "Oh by the way Doctor, our other cat has started meowing in the middle of the night. Why is he doing that?"

You're trying to look up medical recommendations and drug doses in between patient exams, but you can't always find the information you need, and you're constantly being interrupted. The technician working with you today is clearly irritated at your slowness. She doesn't say anything but you can read it in her behavior. She avoids eye contact with you and is doing her best impersonation of Spock from Star Trek, showing no emotion. Yet, you're aware of something simmering under the surface. You're pretty sure you saw her roll her eyes at one of the other technicians when she thought you weren't looking. You wish you could ask her some of the questions you can't ask your boss, but you're convinced she already thinks you're incompetent.

Great, now there's an emergency walk-in! The receptionist carries a small, gray, scruffy dog back to the treatment area. He's been attacked by a larger dog. Your boss is in an exam room with another patient. You have to see the emergency. The dog is laying on his right side. The fur on his left side is soaked with blood. He is having trouble breathing, his gums are pale and his pulses are weak.

You tell the technician to place an intravenous catheter so you can start IV fluids. This dog is clearly in shock. While your tech attempts to place the catheter, you race to the back of the hospital and wheel out the anesthesia machine so you can provide oxygen. You turn on the machine and increase the 02 flow rate while holding the oxygen line in front of the dog's face. You look around for someone else to hold the oxygen line so you can get some injectable pain medicine out of the controlled substances safe, but the entire treatment area is deserted except for you and your technician, and she's still working on the IV catheter. Your boss is still in an exam room.

'Seriously?' you think to yourself, 'no one else in this hospital thinks they should come back to see if we need assistance with this?' You shout towards the front of the clinic hoping someone will hear. "We need some help back here!" After a moment, the receptionist peeks around the corner. She can't physically help since she has to watch the front desk. You tell her to get your boss out of that exam room. "Tell him it's an emergency!" you exclaim.

Your technician has not been able to get an IV catheter in this dog despite shaving both front legs and poking multiple times. The legs are now swollen from the multiple needle stabs which caused blood to leak from the punctured vessels into the adjacent tissues. You're irritated because now neither front leg can be used for a catheter. The technician should have told you she'd blown one leg before ruining the other one! You're going to have to place the IV catheter yourself in one of the back legs.

You hand the oxygen line to your technician and tell her to keep the oxygen flowing towards your patient's mouth and nose. You grab and open a new IV catheter package and then begin shaving the fur over the lateral saphenous vein on the left hind leg. You do a quick alcohol prep – this is no time to be a perfectionist - this dog is dying! You make a conscious effort to ignore the drop of sweat that sprang from your hairline, rolled down your forehead and is now perched atop your right eyebrow. You steady your trembling hand and poke the catheter through the skin. You curse under your breath. Your stomach tightens. There is no flash of blood. You retract and poke again, and again, and again, but you can't hit a vein either.

Finally, your boss enters the treatment area. You are ready for him to rescue you now, but it's too late. The dog has stopped breathing. There's no heartbeat. His eyes are open, staring blankly, his corneas dry and tacky. He's dead.

You wait for your boss to start CPR, but he doesn't. "Shouldn't we start CPR?" you ask, adrenalin gushing through your blood vessels so violently you can hear your own pulse in your eardrums. "No," says your boss calmly as he performs a cursory examination of the dead dog. "We wouldn't be able to fix him even if we did resuscitate him." He walks out of the treatment area and disappears back into the exam room he came from.

Death always brings a unique timbre of silence, especially after an attempt to fight it off has been abandoned. For several moments, you stand there, shaking with disbelief and denial, reliving the sequence of events in your mind and searching for junctures where a different action might have yielded a different result.

You're dubious this had been hopeless from the start. You remember a trauma case you saw on your Emergency Medicine rotation in vet school. It was like being in a movie. You carried the pet into the emergency department and a swarm of technicians, interns and residents immediately went into well-coordinated, purposeful action.

While the intern performed an exam, a technician placed an IV catheter and set up the IV fluid bag and pump, a second technician drew blood and started lab work, and the resident retrieved doses of oxymorphone and a sedative from the safe, injected them, then intubated the patient and started oxygen administration.

Bam! Within five minutes the patient was stabilized. Within twenty minutes there was a diagnosis. The left lung is collapsed! The bite wound punctured her chest wall! It's a tension pneumothorax! She needs a chest tube placed! Call the surgeon! Two hours later the patient was recovering in the ICU.

It's twenty minutes into your lunch hour now but you still have to talk to this dog's owners who are waiting in the lobby. You have to tell them their beloved pet is dead. You couldn't save him. 'That is,' you think to yourself, 'he couldn't be saved under the present circumstances.'

You also have two appointments to finish. One client is still waiting for you to prescribe the medications you said her dog needed for an ear infection, and the other clients are still waiting for you to go over the results of the x-rays you performed on their coughing dog. The receptionist comes back to the treatment area. Her expression is strained.

"The owners of this dog are asking what's going on," she says, "and the people in exam room three are starting to get upset because of the wait."

"Can you tell the people in room three that there's been an emergency, and we're sorry, and I'll be with them as soon as possible?" you ask, hoping she has, in fact, already done this. "I'll talk to this dog's owners right now."

You accompany the dead dog's owners into one of the open exam rooms, closing the door quietly behind you. Their faces show a combination of hope and fear as they look at you expectantly.

"I'm sorry," you say. "He didn't make it."

"She's a *she*!" the wife screeches at you angrily while she collapses, sobbing, into the arms of her husband. He nods at you over her head in understanding.

"Her wounds were too severe," you continue gently.

"Thank you, Doctor," the husband responds with a shaky voice. His nose is red. You can tell he's fighting back tears.

"Is there anything else you'd like to ask me?"

He just closes his eyes and shakes his head, as if speaking again will open the flood gates.

"I am so deeply sorry for your loss," you whisper. "I'll send in the technician to talk about what you'd like to do with her remains."

After exiting the room, you instruct your tech to follow up with them. She tells you that you need to enter your charges into the computer system before she can complete their invoice. You don't want to charge them anything, but you know that's not an option. You remind yourself that when a person dies in a human hospital, their family still gets a bill.

You enter a charge for the emergency fee and oxygen administration, and then enter the prescriptions for your other waiting client. As the prescription labels print, you ask one of the other technicians to fill the medications while you enter exam room three to the sight of two glowering owners. They have been waiting for almost an hour. No one told them what was going on.

By the time you've finished prescribing antibiotics to the coughing Chihuahua for what you're pretty sure is a mild pneumonia, it's time to start afternoon appointments. You grab a candy bar out of your bag and practically swallow it whole, using this same sixty seconds to jot shorthand notes of the important things you need to include in the medical records you still have to write from this morning's appointments.

The remainder of the day unfolds very similarly. You remain behind schedule, slow and pondering, cherry picking what you believe are the most important things to ask your boss. You're not sure if you're imagining it, but you think he might be annoyed with you for constantly bothering him. He is, after all, seeing about four times the number of appointments you are.

How are you ever going to be able to manage a full load of patients when you're failing miserably at seeing so few? Then again, you have noticed your boss taking a few short cuts that you're not sure you approve of. Just a few minutes ago you saw him drawing up a long-acting steroid into a syringe for an itchy cat he was seeing. That appointment only took him ten minutes! You vividly remember one of your vet school professor's derisive comments about this particular treatment. 'Well sure,' you scowl to yourself, 'if we don't take the time to discuss what we really *should* be doing, of course we can see four appointments every hour.'

While your boss ploughs speedily through, you fall further behind every time a technician is unable to draw blood and you have to do it (even though you're quite sure you're not much better at it than they are), every time you have to help restrain a dog for a nail trim because the veterinary assistant is unable to, every time you have to reposition a patient for an x-ray because the technician did it incorrectly the first time.

You've been surprised at how much you needed to supervise the support staff. You're used to being the one being supervised. You were watched like a hawk by the super-techs at the veterinary hospital. You thought you would only have to worry about yourself in this new environment, and that everyone else here would know what they were doing. You actually had to stop one of the technicians from drawing blood on that Chihuahua earlier because she was plunging the full length of a 1 ½ inch needle straight into the little dog's neck.

A vision flashed through your mind of you having to explain to the owner what happened after the dog's trachea or carotid artery was punctured. You're struck by the sudden realization that you not only have to worry about your mistakes but you also have to worry about the mistakes of every technician, veterinary assistant and kennel attendant working under you. Everything is on you. Every error is your responsibility, your reputation, your conscience, your license.

Finally, at the end of the night you get a break. Your last appointment cancels. The chaotic, relentless parade of patients and every snag and unexpected complication that seems to inevitably accompany each one of them is over. You can start writing your medical records and maybe get out of here before 10 o'clock.

You head to the doctors' office and grab your neglected lunch box. Settling into a chair in front of one the computers, it's the first time you've been able to sit down all day. You close your eyes and make your best effort to inhale every oxygen molecule in the room. Then you exhale as slowly as possible, easing into a lower gear as you prepare to write your records. At least now you can eat something and be left in peace for the rest of the night.

You feel your mouth starting to fill up with saliva as you shove half of the tuna fish sandwich you packed this morning into your face and, cheeks bulging, start chewing. It's a dopamine rush. You never imagined a tuna fish sandwich could make you this happy. Then there's a knock at the door. "Come in," you mumble as best you can with your mouth full.

It's your office manager. "Got a couple minutes to talk?" she asks, shutting the door behind her. Your heart sinks. She's going to fire you. Your boss told her you're an incompetent veterinarian. You asked too many stupid questions today. You made too many medical mistakes. One of the clients you saw this morning called to talk to your boss because now their pet is worse. Maybe even dead. Oh God, is it that coughing Chihuahua? "Sure," you answer, trying hard to look nonchalant.

She sits in the chair two desks away and swivels to face you. She leans forward, puts both elbows on her knees, clasps her hands together, and looks at the floor. Her brow is furrowed. You sit up straighter. You stop chewing.

"So," she begins, raising her eyes finally to look at you, "we've had some comments. Several of the staff felt you were harsh with them today. Apparently, they felt you spoke to them in a demeaning way." She pauses, waiting for this to register with you. You search your memory of the whirlwind that was today but can remember nothing about how you might have offended anyone. You were too busy worrying about your patients and your clients.

"Listen," she continues, "I know this was only your first day, and I'm sure it's been stressful for you, but we try really hard here to provide a positive and nurturing environment for the staff. I need you to be more conscious of how you interact with them, okay?"

"Okay," you answer, your mouth still full of shredded fish and Wonder Bread.

After she leaves the room, you realize you're trembling. Your face is hot. Are you having a hot flash? Your mouth, salivating happily just a few moments ago, is now dry. You reach into your lunch box for the can of soda, open it and pour the warm fizzy liquid into your mouth so you can wash the sandwich down. You still have nine records to write but you feel dizzy and your lips and fingertips are tingling. You feel a headache breaking through from behind your eye sockets.

You need to talk to someone about this day - what you saw, what you did, how you felt, what your office manager just said to you. You need to talk to someone right now. You call several of your classmates from veterinary school, one after another, but none of them answer. They're probably having the same kind of day you just had.

You dial home and your mother answers. You want to verbally vomit every single thing you can remember that upset you today. You open your mouth to begin but, realizing the insurmountable gap between what you want to tell her and what she will understand, you say nothing.

"Honey?" your mom says, waiting for you to speak. It turns out you have the ability to mask a hurricane of turbulence in your mind with banal conversation. You tell her you were just calling to confirm your dinner date next Sunday. Are we still on? Yes? Yes, good. Okay. Looking forward to it. See you then. Love you, Mom. Bye.

It's 7:30PM. You have at least two hours of records to write and three client calls to return to answer more questions they had about their visits today. And you have to be back here twelve hours from now. You lean back in the office chair and rub your temples. In vet school, you usually had the luxury of balancing just one or two patients at a time, and because you were "just the student," nobody was depending on you or waiting for you to give them directions. You had a lot of time to look things up and mull things over before anyone even asked for your medical opinion. And that's all it was: An opinion. It could be right or wrong. It made no real difference. If it was right, you'd get kudos from your professor. If it was wrong, you'd learn something.

Today, just eight weeks later, you had to make decisions that could mean the difference between life and death, and you had to make them while juggling multiple patients, appeasing impatient clients, supporting an unsupportive support staff, hiding your terror and frustration, strategically stealing time from a mentor without time to mentor, and ignoring a very loud voice in your head admonishing you for doing things you don't really know how to do.

Transition Shock

As the person inside this story, spend a couple minutes actively cultivating an awareness of how it made you feel emotionally and physically. There's an important reason for this exercise that we'll come to later. For now, just allow yourself to feel everything fully, and consider: What emotions did you feel? What were some of the thoughts going through your mind during this story? What did your body feel like as you were imagining yourself having these experiences? Were there any areas of tension? What was your breathing pattern like? Was your heart rate elevated?

Imagining yourself in this story likely triggered a physiological stress response in your nervous system. Experiencing this on a frequent, ongoing basis is one of the signs that you may be suffering from transition shock. Transition shock results from being thrown into an environment vastly different from what you were prepared for or expecting. The fear of making mistakes, harming patients, and then being discovered to be inept - combines with frustration from feeling unsupported, rushed and forced to provide substandard care while trying to grow into a new role and take on new responsibilities without guidance, a roadmap or even the ability to call a time-out.

You will on occasion feel you have no choice but to practice medicine below what you believe to be the standard of care, despite the ever present fear that an angry client will file a complaint against you with the veterinary board, putting your license at risk. In the longer term, guilt and disillusionment ensue as the ideals espoused in school and in the veterinary teaching hospital must be continually brushed aside due to haste and lack of resources in the real world. A relentless anxiety can develop that will affect every other aspect of your life, from your social interactions to your sleep habits, resulting in serious, long-term psychological and even physical damage.

Transition shock is suspected of being a major contributor to attrition in the field of nursing. It has been estimated that as many as one-third to well over one-half of newly graduated nurses either change jobs or leave the profession completely within their first year out of school, and purportedly, less than 50% of nurses would recommend nursing as a career.[1] This is an eerily similar phenomenon to what seems to be happening in the field of veterinary medicine. Answers to a recent online survey asking veterinarians if they would choose to become vets again given the chance revealed that only 38% of respondents would definitely do so.[20]

The requirement of completing an internship and residency seems to have a mitigating effect on transition shock in doctors who practice human medicine.[1,18] However, as a veterinarian, I had the choice to forego internship and residency and therefore cannot say with any confidence whether they would ease the transition from school to independent practice or not. My suspicion is that the mitigating effects would be highly variable due to the lack of a regulatory body overseeing veterinary internships and a lack of standardization.

Aside from committing to a veterinary internship and residency that may or may not help you avoid the emotional fallout of transition shock, what can be done to prevent an elated, optimistic veterinary graduate from transforming into someone who, just a few years later, may regret becoming a veterinarian altogether?

What You Should Expect

*"Set realistic expectations, and proactively
develop your emotional resiliency."*
- Dr. K

I drove myself relentlessly through years of demanding
undergraduate science classes and hundreds of hours of
working as a veterinary assistant in order to get accepted
into vet school. I mopped the floor of the local ER where I
worked overnights, then fell asleep in Genetics lectures
during the day. Then I drove myself even harder for the
subsequent four years to earn my DVM.

I gained forty pounds in the process. My health
suffered. Friendships I had no time for fell away. My
beloved mother passed away, and my father suffered a
debilitating stroke while I was in veterinary school.

None of this stopped me though because, throughout
those hardships, I held in my mind a vision of myself in
the future as a Doctor of Veterinary Medicine. This vision
of the competent, confident, happy, and fulfilled doctor I
would become once I received my degree sustained and

powered me through all heartbreak to achieve my goal of earning a DVM.

But while I was focusing on manifesting that bright vision, as I stepped from school into practice, all my hopes and ideals were shattered in a high-impact collision with the freight train of transition shock. The vision I had of my future was brighter than any white coat could ever be. I did not have realistic expectations. In order for you to avoid this fate and the emotional wreckage that will ensue, the first thing you need to do is stop focusing on the DVM degree as your goal. Let me explain:

Imagine you're competing in an important foot race that you've trained years for. Let's say this is the "Miss America" or "Mr. Universe" of all foot races. You represent your home state, having outrun every other competitor from your state in previous races. Now the race is between the best runners from every state in the nation.

Your family and friends, who've been so supportive through the years of intensive training and competitions, are in the crowd of rowdy, cheering spectators. Your heart is pounding in your head while you wait, crouched in starting position behind the black and white checkered starting line. You need to remain focused to achieve your top performance so you do your best to ignore the screaming crowd, as well as the breathing and fidgeting of the other runners surrounding you. You crook your neck to raise your eyes and level them at the track ahead. It is four miles to the finish line.

The race official yells, "Ready, set, go!" You use the powerful muscles in your legs to explode over the starting line. You quickly reach your optimum rhythm where the frequency of your feet pounding the ground is synchronized with the counterbalancing swing of your arms. You have practiced this run countless times and you know exactly how hard you can push yourself to achieve the right balance between the speed required to stay ahead of your competitors and the endurance needed to reach the finish line.

You are momentarily distracted by the strength of your competitors though. You're used to pulling ahead of other runners right away, but these people are keeping up with you! You decide to ignore the encroaching figures in your peripheral vision and focus instead on the track ahead and the sound of your own breathing. In through the nose, out through the mouth. In, out, in, out; you're like a powerful machine revving itself up to maximum power. By sheer force of will you manage to pull more energy up from the deepest reserves within and propel yourself ahead of the other runners.

After half an hour of this, fountains of perspiration are bursting from every sweat gland and combining into rivulets that stream down your cheeks, your nose, your arms and legs. You feel no shortness of breath but a numbing heaviness is starting to develop in your legs. Your body is tiring. Half a mile to go. You are still ahead of all the other runners.

Keep going! Don't slow down! You can do it! There! You can see the finish line! You're going to make it! You're going to win! Now you can use that last burst of energy to power through the ribbon stretched across the track.

You reach your hands high above your head in victory as the ribbon hits your chest. People are cheering. Photos are being snapped. Someone throws a bucket of cold water over you and pats you on the back. Your soaked shirt makes a sloshing sound with each congratulatory slap.

"Excuse me, folks," the race official's voice booms over the PA system. "Folks! Listen up, listen up, please!"

The noise of the crowd subsides to a low frequency buzz and the official continues. "It has been decided, due to the significance of this race and the exceptionally high caliber of all the contestants, that effective as of now, the finish line is to be moved, increasing the total distance in this race from four to nine miles."

Wait, what? Now that you've expended the last of your energy to win a four mile race, you have to continue racing on another course that is just as long - plus one more mile?! While it is true that you're an exceptionally high caliber runner, and you probably can run another five miles, in your present state of physical exhaustion plus the emotional combination of shock and outrage, how great do you think you're going to feel when you reach the "real" finish line?

What if you had known before you started that this would happen? What if you knew, even back when you first started training years ago, that the real distance in this race wasn't going to be four miles, as everyone was saying, but nine. Would that have changed your strategy? Would you have trained differently? Raced differently?

If you continue to think of earning a DVM as your goal, you will end up feeling just like the runner in this story at the end of that race. You will do much better in the long run by readjusting your focus to a finish line on a more distant horizon. I'm going to tell you something now that may be difficult for you to swallow, but it's the truth. It's the red pill that Neo chose over the blue pill in the film *The Matrix*. It's the realistic expectation you need to have now in order to avoid disillusionment later. Are you ready? Here it is:

> *Genuine transformation of student to doctor*
> *will take <u>five years more</u> than merely*
> *earning the right to be called Doctor.*

Veterinarians in their <u>first five years </u>of practice report the highest levels of psychological distress and job dissatisfaction, and are more likely to report they are unhappy and that they regret their career choice.[14] Consider this in tandem with Malcom Gladwell's assertion that the minimum number of hours required to achieve mastery in any discipline is ten thousand. Ten thousand hours equates to <u>five years </u>of practicing as a full-time veterinarian.

I don't believe this five year parallel between the time it takes to feel better *about yourself* as a practicing veterinarian, and the time it takes to feel better *about being a veterinarian* is a coincidence. Although you won't be a "Master" after five years, you will have seen and done enough to *feel* like a real doctor, and you cannot enjoy *being* a doctor, until you *feel* like a doctor. The trick is to get through those difficult first five years after veterinary school with your emotional health intact.

Why Doctors Need Emotional Resiliency

I have always been a highly reactive person. I could go from perfectly content to raging mad in less than a single breath. People have said things to me like, "your elevator doesn't stop anywhere in between the bottom and the top floor, does it?"And quite frankly, no, it didn't. As far as I was concerned, the middle ground didn't exist, since I had never been there. Up until becoming a veterinarian, I still managed to do pretty well despite my reactive nature. Sure, I experienced stress, I got upset, I even suffered from mild depression once in a while when exhausted by my own swinging moods, but it was different. It never affected my ability to function and I never considered suicide.

I used to work in what many consider one of the most stressful industries there is: Corporate advertising. I was an account executive on the worldwide IBM account at Ogilvy & Mather, one of the top advertising agencies in the world. The stress in advertising stems largely from the non-negotiable material submission deadlines of various media, like television stations, magazines and newspapers.

If you missed a deadline, the money your client paid for the media space was forfeited, and you lost your job. If clients requested changes, or corrections needed to be made to the materials before submission, the time those changes took varied depending on the complexity of the material, the art director or copywriter on your team, and how many other jobs were making their way through the production department.

We were one hour to a magazine deadline one day when my assistant came to me wearing a look of cringing apology and bouncing in place on her toes to signal the need for desperate hurry. She told me the art director was refusing to sign off on the final materials we needed to send to the magazine. This art director was known for being a bit of a fussbudget.

I stormed into his office to confront him and learned the reason for his refusal was that he didn't want to sign his name on anything he felt was subpar, and the left margin of the ad was 2 millimeters off. At this point we had less than an hour to deliver the materials to the magazine. There wasn't enough time to get the production department to fix this error. He had to sign off. No diplomatic reasoning could persuade him to tarnish his perfect reputation by signing his name to something imperfect. I literally had to scream at him to get him to sign off on that magazine ad.

As I exited the art director's office, trembling with rage, a colleague by the name of Michael approached and put his hands on my shoulders to calm me. Michael knew what it felt like to be under great pressure. The week prior he had screamed, "Because I told you to do it that way!" so loudly at his administrative assistant that everyone on the 7th floor heard it. Then, he pushed her desk over, sending its contents sprawling across the floor.

Michael looked deep into my eyes now, and with great empathy, softly said, "Remember, nobody dies." I chuckled then. I shook my head as I smiled at him and said, "You're right. Thank you." Then the rage dissipated and I was fine. We all went out for drinks later that night and had a good laugh over what happened. I wish someone could help me snap out of a bad mood by reminding me that "nobody dies" in veterinary medicine, but we all know that's not true.

After I graduated and started working as an ER veterinarian, my first mentor told me that good judgment comes from experience, and experience comes from bad judgment. In medicine, there are many things you can only learn on your feet, in the weeds and at your patients' expense. Every doctor has their own "pile of bones." Every doctor will make mistakes that harm or even kill the patients they are trying to help. Even doctors with decades of experience make mistakes because medicine is not a perfect science, and because we are human beings. However, you are most likely to commit the majority of your worst mistakes in your first five years of practice.

I remember my first critical case. I was one month out of vet school and had just moved back to Chicago to help look after my aging father. I was incredibly fortunate to have been hired right away as a full-time ER veterinarian at a well equipped emergency and specialty center north of the city. The night an old black cat I'll call Shadow was carried into the ER, I was working my way through day three of being a real live practicing veterinarian.

Shadow was very sick. He could not stand or even lift his head, though he was conscious and aware. He was dehydrated, weak, and old. There was a palpable mass in his abdomen. His blood work revealed that he was in severe kidney failure, and he was no longer urinating, which made his prognosis much worse.

I knew from my vet school lectures and reading in nephrology that my medical objective was to rehydrate Shadow and to do everything I could to get him to urinate. If he could not be made to urinate, there was no hope for him short of kidney dialysis, and owners of very sick, old cats who are able or willing to spend many thousands of dollars on kitty kidney dialysis are few and far between.

But I was missing the point. It isn't enough to know what medically needs to be done. One must consider whether or not it should be done. What are the chances that the appropriate medical treatment will lead to a successful outcome? Can this patient be saved? If he can, what will his life look like after you save it? Even if I'd had the mind to ask then, I couldn't have correctly answered those questions about Shadow that night because I lacked the experience, and the judgment.

Shadow had an intravenous and a urinary catheter placed in him. He spent the next several hours lying recumbent on a towel in a cage in an unfamiliar place surrounded by bright lights, beeping fluid pumps, barking dogs, and by people who cared for him, but didn't know him and didn't love him. His owners had gone home believing, as I had believed when I told them, that there was a chance we could pull him through.

As the hours of intravenous fluid therapy failed to improve his status, I started administering injections of medications meant as last ditch efforts to get him to urinate. (I now know it was too early to expect Shadow to urinate. He was still far too dehydrated.)

He vocalized with a sad yowling sound after each injection. I don't know whether the injections caused him physical discomfort or whether he was delusional or whether he was trying to tell me that he had had enough and wanted to die, so I went on trying to save him.

As my shift that night was coming to an end, I turned over my hospitalized patients, including Shadow, to the overnight veterinarian who, I was told, euthanized Shadow shortly after I left. Yes, it hurt my pride to hear that from the technicians. But the truth is, that veterinarian did the right thing. It's what I should have done for Shadow eight hours earlier, while his owners were there, so they could have held him in their arms, and so he could have passed peacefully, feeling loved and safe. My naiveté and hubris robbed Shadow and his owners of something they should have had, and could have had, if only they had seen a different doctor that night.

Retrospectively, it seems obvious to me that Shadow's kidney values were too high, his electrolytes were too imbalanced, his clinical presentation was too critical, and he was too old for us to realistically expect to restore any reasonable quality of life to him, especially in light of the mass in his abdomen, which was probably what caused his clinical decline.

But as a new doctor who hadn't yet unpacked everything she'd learned in vet school, and who hadn't yet built any bridges between the separate, discrete medical folders in her mind, all I could see was a cat in kidney failure. The experience I gained from my bad judgment on Shadow's case was helpful to me, but the cost was Shadow's prolonged suffering, and my ongoing remorse and shame. Remorse because I know so clearly now what I didn't know then, and because I did something I wish I hadn't that I can't go back and change. Shame because it was my hubris that drove me to do it. Three days as a practicing veterinarian and I was utterly convinced I could save him. I was convinced I could save anyone.

A career in veterinary medicine is filled with valuable lessons like this. I have many more stories of patients I've failed and lessons I've learned from those failures. The more memorable the lesson, the more valuable the learning experience - the higher the emotional cost. Hippocrates said something like, "The art of medicine is long, and life is short." I think what he meant was that medicine never runs out of things to teach us.

You too will make mistakes. You will make them because your medical knowledge was imperfect. You will make them because you were incapable of juggling so many patients at once. You will make them because you were concentrating too hard on your own performance instead of properly supervising your support staff. You will make them because you were distracted by multiple people asking you endless questions throughout your shift. You will make them because you were trying too hard, because you were tired, because you were over confident, because you were nervous, because you were in a hurry, because you were upset. Sometimes patients will die and you won't know whether it was your fault or not, but you will come up with dozens of explanations for how it might have been.

If you're like most people who have their sights set on veterinary school, you're probably used to succeeding because you strive for perfection in everything you do, and you tend to be very hard on yourself for every mistake and perceived failure. This is both your blessing and your curse. This hard-driving, perfectionist quality will serve you well as you prepare for and proceed through veterinary school, where the rules are clear and all the players have well defined roles; where every question has one right answer, and there is a logical and predictable correlation between how hard you work and how well you do as a student. However, this same perfectionist quality will be your undoing in the messy reality that awaits you in your years after veterinary school.

If you have worked or volunteered at a veterinary hospital, you may have already overheard one doctor saying to another, "Never forget your pile of bones." What they mean is: Never forget what you learned from the patients you harmed. These are unavoidable and necessary but profoundly painful lessons. More painful for perfectionists who beat themselves up for even the smallest errors. More painful still for the compassionate person who became a veterinarian to help animals.

If you are a compassionate perfectionist, I can say unequivocally that you are the best person for this job. No one else is going to drive themselves harder to do better for their patients. No one is going to be harder on you than you are on yourself for every single mistake you make. Over the course of your first five years in practice, that compassionate perfectionism is going to make you into an amazing clinician.

But – and this is very important, especially if you already know yourself to be prone to depression or anxiety - unless you can learn to accept the imperfections of practice, unless you can learn to be patient with your own shortcomings, unless you can learn to forgive yourself, and to learn from your mistakes without becoming emotionally crushed by the accumulating weight on your conscience - even though you may be the best person for this job, this isn't going to be the best job for you. Without the emotional resilience you need, you will end up fatigued, burned out, regretful of your career choice, and most likely, chronically depressed long before you cross that finish line at five years of full-time practice.

Resistance is... Not in Your Best Interest

Most sources of advice on preventing or treating the negative emotional toll that clinical practice can inflict include the same list of oft-repeated recommendations: Meditate, do some deep breathing, practice gratitude, etcetera. Perhaps it's because by the time I was exposed to these ideas I was already emotionally compromised, but to me these suggestions just seemed glib.

I felt I'd already been down that road when I explored New Age Spiritualism. Long before I decided to become a veterinarian, I sought enlightenment and emotional balance by reading books like *The Celestine Prophecy* and *The Tenth Insight* and various titles by Shakti Gawain. I wore Reiki healing bracelets made of rose quartz and Chakra healing bracelets made of volcanic lava. I burned cinnamon incense to enhance my personal power, amber for wisdom, rain for healing and relaxation.

But this quest to understand the universe and find my peace within it was fruitless. I felt no closer to understanding life, and my elevator still didn't stop anywhere between the bottom and tops floors. Because of this past failure, I was cynical and turned off by the fluffy, new-age language and culture that seemed to accompany words like *meditation* and *gratitude*. I felt I'd found the enlightenment I'd sought in the hard sciences, and now that I had the concrete and sensible answers I'd been looking for, I was not going to be persuaded by promises of unquantifiable benefits like achieving a state of Zen or harmonizing my chakras.

As a veterinarian, when contemplating meditation, I imagined myself as Lieutenant Worf in the Star Trek Next Generations *Cost of Living* episode where he reluctantly stews in a mud bath and sneers, "You're just supposed to sit here?" I felt similarly skeptical about practicing gratitude ("Hello, nice to meet you. My name is Pollyanna!") and developing hobbies ("I don't know everything I need to know and I'm six months behind on reading my medical journals as it is! Medicine is my life now. I don't have time for hobbies!").

Time is not something a busy practicing vet is willing to waste, and without confidence that the time invested in these activities would yield concrete benefits, I felt the only solution available to me was to hide my emotional reactivity and headbutt my way through adversity as I'd always done before. On the outside, I appeared to be coping adequately with the strains and stresses of practicing veterinary medicine. On the inside, I was using an ice pick to stab myself in my chest and in my abdomen each time a patient got worse instead of better, each time I failed to practice perfect medicine because I was unable to triumph over the limited resources at my hospital, or the limited resources of my clients, or my own inadequate knowledge and skills.

It didn't take long for these self-inflicted emotional traumas to deplete me of the power I'd depended on in the past to bounce back. The depression and anxiety I developed during my early years of practice was quite a different animal from anything I'd encountered before. It devoured me, and all my remaining energy went to struggling to subsist in the dark gullet of this wicked creature that I couldn't escape. I lost hope that my life as a veterinarian would ever be anything but the pit of misery and angst it had become, and for the first time in my life, death began to look like the only plausible way out.

Once you get to a place like this, even if you manage to claw your way out, you'll still remember every stab to your chest and abdomen in vivid detail. You can't erase emotional trauma like that out of your brain. I know veterinarians who, like myself, feel full up with traumatic memories that haunt them for years, that come up from the past out of context and plunge them into guilt and despair. I was running on the treadmill the other day and for no reason that I can think of suddenly found myself remembering a euthanasia I regretted from three years in the past. I immediately started sobbing so hard I fell to my knees and couldn't continue my run. This is what it's like to have post-traumatic stress disorder (PTSD).

Some may take offense at comparing the emotional

trauma of veterinarians to PTSD, the diagnosis most commonly associated with soldiers. I'm sure, like any pathology, there's a spectrum, with the PTSD of soldiers being at the far end of the curve. A soldier who has seen battle may consider the emotional traumas veterinarians experience insignificant, and perhaps by comparison, they are. But the cumulative effect of these daily "insignificant" emotional traumas can cause the same symptoms of PTSD - hyper-arousal, hyper-vigilance, flashbacks, depression, anxiety, difficulty sleeping, avoidance - so I say, if it looks like a duck, and it quacks like a duck, then it's a duck.

One of the bedrock principles I learned in vet school was that some injuries, for instance, trauma to a knee or ankle severe enough to require surgical intervention, can never truly be fixed. Surgery may help make the joint functional again, but it cannot restore the perfect alignment that existed before the trauma occurred. Ideal function will not be regained. There will always be some degree of pain. The joint will be more vulnerable to re-injury, and the anatomical derangement, however subtle, can lead to deleterious changes in other associated structures in the body.

PTSD is like this. It can never truly be cured. The psychological traumas cannot be forgotten. The skin that grows over the old wounds will remain forever fragile, and the disorder can affect every other aspect of one's emotional life. Once it develops, the underlying psychic anatomy becomes irreparably altered, and the best one can hope for is to learn to effectively manage the symptoms.

While I did claw my way out of that depression, I found I was even more emotionally reactive than I had been before. The hyper-vigilance of my irreparably altered psychic anatomy increased my vulnerability to falling back into the pit I'd worked so hard to escape. I knew that, unless I found an effective way to deal with the pressures of practice, I would succumb again. So I started searching the medical literature for information on how doctors could maintain their own psychological wellbeing. Surely, there had to be recommendations that were grounded on sound scientific evidence.

That's when I found the article about transition shock, and from there, in some random but fortuitous process, I managed to find one academic article after another demonstrating the quantifiable efficacy of practices like meditation and gratitude. More importantly for me, these articles explained in materialistic, scientific terms why and how these things work. It's the mechanistic explanation and scientific evidence of the benefits of these practices that changed my attitude toward them, and inspired me to give them an honest try.

Through these practices, I've discovered that the middle ground between my bottom and top floors actually does exist. I've visited this place. When I'm there, I can shut out unhelpful traumatic memories, I can talk myself out of anxiety and the kind of ruminations that lead to depression, and I can reframe the vicissitudes of being a veterinarian, and of life in general, into opportunities for learning and growth. When I perform these practices daily, I'm able to spend most of my time in this place of emotional balance. If I skip even one day, however, it becomes difficult to find my way back to that middle ground. If I skip several days, I start to forget this place exists at all.

If I had known how to find this place of emotional balance before, I wouldn't have wounded myself over and over again as I did. I would have had the resilience to better weather the emotional storms of my first five years in practice, and I wouldn't have to work so hard now to maintain my psychological wellbeing. You don't have to make the same mistake I did. You can use these practices to proactively build the emotional resilience that can help you get through those harrowing first five years of practice without developing the emotional complications I, and so many of my colleagues, have.

Do not underestimate the stress you're going to experience as a veterinarian. Research indicates it is much more difficult to master these practices when under emotional duress.[17] I can personally attest to this. Olympian athletes train, on average, eight years in advance of The Games.[19] Likewise, if you are serious about becoming the best veterinarian you can be, you must begin training years in advance as well, not only intellectually, as with the required science prerequisites, but also emotionally.

Why it Works – a Scientific Explanation

Holocaust survivor, psychiatrist and author of the best-selling book *Man's Search for Meaning*, Viktor Frankl said, "Between stimulus and response there is a space. In that space is our power to choose our response." Everything I'm going to recommend really boils down to just one thing: Expanding the space between stimulus and response.

We may not be able to control what happens to us (the stimulus), but we can learn to control how we respond, and almost invariably, it is our response that determines the trajectory of how our lives unfold after an incident, not the incident itself. The word "response" may conjure images of a verbal or physical reaction, such as those typically directed at an object or a person outside ourselves. However, "response" can also refer to how we react internally.

The more expansive our stimulus-response space, the greater the variety of possible responses we have to choose from, and the greater our power to choose a response that mitigates, rather than exacerbates, an adverse event. I often think of this space as a period of time. It can be as a short as a fraction of a second, in which case our response is going to be purely instinctive. Or it can be infinitely long, if we have cultivated sufficient self-control.

I also find it helpful to think of the stimulus-response space as an actual, physical space; one that offers more choices when it's big and fewer choices when it's small - like a travel hub. An expanded stimulus-response space can hold as many choices as New York's JFK International Airport, with hundreds of possible destinations available. On the other hand, a narrow stimulus-response space is akin to the tiny airport where I live in Flagstaff, Arizona. From this airport there is only one place you can go and that's Phoenix, Arizona. A narrow stimulus-response space has one option, and no choice.

Earlier in this book I mentioned that the limbic system is the emotional part of the brain. Within the limbic system is a structure called the amygdala. The amygdala is like a switchboard in the emotional part of the brain. It's the gatekeeper of our stimulus-response space. It assigns emotional meaning to every event and situation.

If the amygdala interprets an event or situation in a negative or threatening way, it will trigger a stress response in the autonomic nervous system, the part of our nervous system over which we have no conscious control. When the stress response is triggered, adrenaline and cortisol begin coursing through the circulatory system. Heart rate and blood-pressure increase. Breathing becomes fast and shallow. Most importantly, connections to the cerebral cortex, the thinking part of the brain, are short-circuited. [2,9,17]

The amygdala triggered stress response inhibits our ability to think,[5] narrowing our stimulus-response space and preventing us from responding in creative and productive ways. The result is an almost instantaneous, instinctive, knee-jerk response of the fight-or-flight variety. Negative emotions shunt us away from the JFK Airport part of our brain and toward the part of our brain that's more like the tiny airport in Flagstaff, Arizona, where only one destination is possible.

Unfortunately, most of us have an amygdala that is inherently predisposed to interpret the world in a negative light. As psychologist Rick Hansen explains in his Huffington Post blogpost entitled, *Confronting the Negativity Bias*, "The alarm bell of your brain — the amygdala […]— uses about two-thirds of its neurons to look for bad news: it's primed to go negative." This negativity bias makes perfect sense when considered in evolutionary terms. It increases the chances of survival in life-or-death situations.

Imagine yourself as a young teenager three million years in the past. You are of the early hominid genus Australopithecus. You are walking happily along with your friend, another Australopithecus, in an African woodland. You and your friend have been walking for many hours and you're getting hungry.

To your delight, you spy a large bush beside the trail that is covered in plump, ripe berries. You and your friend eagerly begin picking the berries and popping them in your mouths. They burst with sweet flavor on your tongue. Your stomach growls with hunger and you and your friend set your minds to eating every last berry on this bush, but then a saber toothed cat appears. Is it in your best interest to focus on the positive (delicious, ripe, plump berries) or the negative (saber toothed cat)?

Lucky for you, your grandfather was a skittish creature who was always the first to flee at any sign of danger, and you inherited his reactive amygdala. The moment you see the big cat, you experience a rush of frantic energy and begin running away as fast as your skinny legs will carry you.

Your friend however, a descendent of one of the more easy going people in your tribe, thought he had time to stuff just a few more berries in his mouth and still get away. Which one of you survives and gets to grow up and have children of his own? Which one of you passes the genes of your ancestors on to future generations?

We human beings who exist today are distant descendants of the Australopith who focused on the saber-toothed cat instead of the delicious, plump berries. We inherited his genes, his negatively primed amygdala, his predisposition to negativity, and his narrow stimulus-response space. These things have granted a survival advantage to every surviving hominid descendant up to the advent of modern civilization.

The good news is, in modern civilization, you are statistically unlikely to ever find yourself in a life-or-death situation. The bad news is, your amygdala doesn't know this. The same instinctive, knee-jerk responses that would have continued to serve us well, arguably even up to the Industrial Revolution, are paradoxically counterproductive today.

In that African woodland, three million years ago, an instinctive response to a negatively perceived situation or event would look like someone running or fighting for their lives. In today's "polite society," (such as the veterinary hospital where you'll begin your career) it's more likely to look like a snarky word, or a defensive argument, or a self-flagellating sigh, or... Nothing.

Despite the fact a stress response has been triggered, our hearts may be racing, and we may be very upset internally, in polite society, we hide as much of that as we are able. Hidden though they may be, these negative thoughts and emotions trigger a negativity cascade that continues to affect our thinking and behavior long after the perceived threat has passed.

When we allow our amygdala to interpret an event or situation in a negative way, we fall by default into a tiny stimulus-response space where the instinctive reaction to a perceived negative situation or event is a negative emotion. If we react outwardly from this negative emotion, even if our reactions are subtle, there may be social or professional repercussions. We will likely interpret those repercussions negatively as well, and a vicious cycle of negativity begins.

Even if we succeed in hiding our negative emotional or mental reactions, those thoughts and emotions continue to exist in our minds where they fuel negative beliefs about ourselves and the world. These negative thoughts behave like prions in the brain – those pernicious proteins that cause Mad Cow Disease. They distort everything they come into contact with. Negative thoughts beget negative thoughts. This cascade leads to the path of rumination and social withdrawal, creating another vicious cycle of negativity.

The more often a negative emotional response happens in our brains, the more likely it is to keep on happening. Just as frequent traffic over the same path in the woods creates a trail others are more likely to follow, the neural pathway for negativity in our brains becomes easier to activate the more often it's activated. Under conditions of adversity and stress, such as your first five years after veterinary school, a self-perpetuating "negative emotional spiral" can ensue, leading to depression, chronic anxiety or other types of mental and physical illnesses.[5] This is why, in this day and age, these instinctive, knee jerk responses are more likely to cause us harm than save our lives.

There is something we can do about it though. This is where my favorite part of the brain, the thinking brain, finally takes center stage. The late, great astrophysicist and author Carl Sagan said, "Deep inside the skull of every one of us there is something like a brain of a crocodile. Surrounding the R-complex is the limbic system or mammalian brain, which evolved tens of millions of years ago in ancestors who were mammal but not yet primates. It is a major source of our moods and emotions, of our concern and care for the young. And finally, on the outside, living in uneasy truce with the more primitive brains beneath, is the cerebral cortex; civilization is a product of the cerebral cortex."

So it follows that we must master the powers of the cerebral cortex to thrive in civilization. The largest portion of the cerebral cortex is the neocortex. "Neo" means new. It's the most recently evolved part of our brain. Even though the amygdala is an ancient structure in our brain with hard to break habits, we don't have to let it determine our moods, our emotional responses, or our destiny. We now know that the emotional pathways of the brain can be rewired using the cerebral cortex to control emotional experience.[31]

Certain kinds of psychotherapy as well as meditation, both of which exemplify active uses of the cerebral cortex, have been shown to beneficially affect not only the function of the amygdala but even its structure.[2,12,17] In essence, we can use our newer, thinking brain to retrain, and possibly even reshape, our older, emotional brain.[10] With conscious, direct effort, we can expand the stimulus-response space and transform our caveman (or woman) amygdala into a less reactive organ.

In her 2001 article in the journal *American Psychologist*, Barbara Fredrickson also calls attention to the narrowing effect of negative emotions. She uses the term "momentary thought-action repertoire" which, for all intents and purposes related to the scope of this book, is perfectly analogous to the stimulus-response space. The question she posed in her research was: If negative emotions narrow our "momentary thought-action repertoire," do positive emotions have the opposite effect? While she was Professor of Psychology at the University of Michigan, Fredrickson performed multiple, well designed experiments confirming that indeed "certain discrete positive emotions – including joy, interest, contentment, pride, and love […] all share the ability to broaden people's momentary thought-action repertoires […]"[4]

Importantly, Fredrickson's research also demonstrated that the effects of experiencing positive emotions are cumulative, adding up over time, and "outlasting the transient emotional states." This means that, even if we are not in a positive state at the moment we confront an adverse event or situation, if we have actively cultivated sufficient positive emotions in advance, our stimulus-response space will have been sufficiently expanded to enable a controlled, thoughtful and creative response. Thus, the negativity cascade can be thwarted.

How do positive emotions expand the stimulus-response space? Think of it this way: The amygdala's job is to keep us alive by vigilantly watching for danger. Every time the negativity cascade gets triggered, the amygdala becomes more convinced it's living in a dangerous world. It becomes more reactive. The more reactive the amygdala becomes, the smaller the stimulus-response space becomes.

But if we purposefully cultivate an abundance of

positive feelings such as joy, love and curiosity, and if we can learn to use the powers of the cerebral cortex to prevent negativity cascades, not only will we be capable of responding in creative and productive ways in the moment, we will also be sending signals to our amygdala that we are safe, and eventually, it will learn to relax. This is the underlying, scientific justification for meditation, gratitude and other practices recommended in the next section.

Recommended Practices

I've compiled a set of seven practices to help you proactively develop emotional resiliency. They'll serve you best if used together and practiced regularly and you'll benefit most if you begin these practices with an already healthy state of mind. If you are currently suffering from depression, anxiety or other emotional or psychological challenges, depending on the severity of your affliction, these alone may not be sufficient to help, and you should seek the professional and medical advice of a psychiatrist.

While you could follow these recommendations to the letter and benefit, the ideal strategy for fostering and maintaining emotional wellbeing is going to be different for all of us. My hope is that by introducing these practices to you, you'll be inspired to do your own research. Experiment for yourself to find the regimen that works best for you. The important thing is to begin now, and to maintain a regular practice to support the on-going cultivation and maintenance of your own emotional resilience.

Thwarting the Negativity Cascade

When I talk about a negativity cascade, I'm usually referring not only to the initial negative interpretation and reaction, but also to any further repercussions that may ensue, whether internal or external. Here however, I'd like to just focus on the initial reaction, because this is where prevention and intervention do the greatest good.

I'm going to start by dissecting and naming the three major steps of the negativity cascade. Each of the recommended practices targets a different step in the cascade. Let's use an example from the imaginary story about your first day as a doctor. Remember when your practice manager told you that some of the other employees complained about you? Below is a likely sequence for the negativity cascade that would follow:

1: Emotional interpretation by amygdala >
2: Negative emotional interpretation >
3: Stress response

Can you remember how you felt when you imagined yourself inside that story? How quickly did the sequence above unfold? My guess is you experienced the entire cascade as if it were one, instantaneous reaction. That's how it feels when we react from a narrow stimulus-response space, as most of us are prone to do.

What the following recommended practices can help you do is to expand your stimulus-response space so that you can experience the negativity cascade in slow motion, giving your cerebral cortex the opportunity to intervene at specific junctures to either thwart the cascade or abbreviate the stress response. The earlier in the cascade you can intervene, the easier it is to stop.

Step 1: Emotional Interpretation

This is the intercept point with the biggest bang for your buck. <u>This *is* the stimulus-response space</u>. It's the point *before* your amygdala has assigned negative emotional meaning to something. It's the point at which all possible response options remain open and available to you. You're in JFK International Airport baby, and your pockets are full of money. You can go anywhere you wish. Paris, France? Sydney, Australia? How about Tokyo, Japan? If you can train your brain to override its natural predisposition to negative emotional interpretation, you'll be quite unflappable. Adversity will be nothing more than an opportunity to innovate and find creative solutions. The following five practices can help you directly expand your stimulus-response space.

> **PRACTICE #1**: Loving-Kindness Meditation (LKM)
>
> **RATIONALE**: People with PTSD arguably have the most narrow stimulus-response spaces. Because of the severity and/or frequency of traumatic experiences in their past (some of which actually may have been genuine life-or-death situations), their amygdalae are hypervigilant and hyper-reactive.
>
> A 2013 pilot study using LKM to treat veterans with PTSD demonstrated a significant

improvement in their symptoms of PTSD after 12 weeks. An increase in self-compassion was attributed as the mediating factor.[11] A 2011 literature review of Loving Kindness and Compassion meditation noted "self-compassion moderates reactions to distressing events" and "individuals with high levels of self-compassion reported less negative emotion when confronting real, imagined or remembered negative events." Analysis of the literature revealed that LKM increases self-compassion and "led to shifts in peoples' daily experiences of a wide range of positive emotions."[7] A 2015 systematic review of 342 papers on Loving Kindness and Compassion Meditation found significant increases in positive moods and positive thinking, and significant decreases in negative moods and psychological distress.[16]

Similar positive results have been found in people practicing mindfulness meditation. However, I'm recommending LKM instead for two reasons. First, most beginners (myself included) find great difficulty trying to clear their minds of all thoughts by focusing only on their breathing, which is what mindfulness meditation asks you to do. LKM is a meditation where you're intentionally thinking *something*, and therefore I believe it to be a better and less discouraging practice for beginners.

Second, there is no more important trait for a future veterinarian to cultivate than self-compassion. In her book *Lovingkindness: The Revolutionary Art of Happiness,* Sharon Salzberg tells us, "Love for others without the foundation of love for ourselves becomes a loss of boundaries [...]." This is the gateway to negativity via guilt, inappropriate self-sacrifice and resentment. I have seen this happen to myself and to other veterinarians, and I can think of no other profession where the self-compassion required to maintain healthy boundaries is more essential. In order to successfully cultivate positive emotions in ourselves, we must first believe we are worthy.

Another benefit of meditating on a regular basis, whether you use LKM or mindfulness or some other kind of meditation, is the ability you'll develop to observe your own thoughts, and to recognize that you are not your thoughts. You are the thinker behind the thoughts. You don't have to react to or believe them. You can question them, find them curious, interesting. As Sam Harris says in his book, *Waking Up*, "That which is aware of sadness is not sad. That which is aware of fear in not fearful." Regular meditation over time will grant you the power to take the perspective of the thinker of the thoughts, at any moment. When you can do that, the size and duration of the stimulus-response space is completely under your control.

INSTRUCTIONS: LKM can be practiced anytime, anywhere and in any position - sitting, lying down, even walking. Try just fifteen minutes of LKM every day. The standard Loving Kindness Meditation protocol is to repeat some variation of the following sentences (you can personalize and vary the phrases as you wish): *"May you be safe, may you enjoy physical happiness, may you enjoy mental happiness, may your life be filled with ease and contentment."*

The idea is to speak or think these phrases while you direct thoughts of benevolent compassion to a series of subjects. Typically, you begin the meditation by directing these phrases towards yourself, then at a benefactor or mentor, then toward a well loved friend or family member, then at a neutral person - like the clerk at the post office or local convenience store, then at an enemy or some difficult person in your life, and finally to every living being everywhere. To avoid distraction, don't choose subjects for whom you have sexual feelings.

Because sending loving kindness toward ourselves is difficult for many of us, you can instead begin the meditation by imagining yourself surrounded by everyone (people and pets too) who loves or has ever loved you. Picture them sending loving kindness to you, rather than trying to send loving kindness to yourself. Feel yourself receiving their loving kindness and filling up with it so that you can then send it to others.

The second most common challenge in this meditation is sending loving kindness to an enemy or difficult person. The first time I tried, I felt a very strong mental resistance. I pushed through it by merely repeating the words as I thought of the person, even though I felt no loving kindness. Interestingly, after the first repetition (I usually repeat the four phrases four times for each subject), I found myself imagining the possible personal struggles and sorrows this person might have faced in their life that caused them to behave in a hurtful way towards me. After that, I had little trouble with this part of the meditation. I've also noticed that even when I'm not meditating, thinking about this person no longer inspires anger. Now, when I meet someone who's being cantankerous or rude (you will encounter plenty of this as a veterinarian), I try to think to myself, 'you're the difficult person I'm going to send loving-kindness to the next time I meditate!' This has the potential to instantly stop a negativity cascade in my brain.

PRACTICE #2: Gratitude

RATIONALE: Of all the positive emotions, gratitude appears to have the strongest correlation with emotional resilience. Perhaps it's because, like self-compassion, gratitude enhances our ability to enjoy other positive emotions.[8] It's much easier to experience feelings of happiness and love when we actively acknowledge the good things in our lives. Additionally, gratitude appears to decrease the frequency and potency of negative emotions by helping us to interpret adverse events in terms of how we may learn and grow from them.

Interestingly, gratitude also appears to help people suffering from PTSD. A 2006 study on Vietnam veterans showed an inverse correlation between feelings of gratitude and symptoms of PTSD. In other words, the more gratitude a veteran reported feeling, the less likely they were to suffer from PTSD.[13]

INSTRUCTIONS: Practice gratitude daily by doing the following three things:

1. Throughout your day, be always on the lookout for good things and relish them in the moment you find them. For instance, if you're walking down the street and a passing stranger smiles and

nods, rather than reflexively smiling back then resuming your thoughts about the train you need to catch or a project at work you're concerned about, take a few seconds to acknowledge and appreciate the gesture of friendliness as the gift that it is. If your morning coffee is wonderfully aromatic, take the time to notice and feel grateful for the pleasant sensation. If the clouds in the sky have formed an especially stunning pattern, notice and be grateful that you are there to witness such beauty. There are hundreds of good things to be found in every one of our days, if we look for them.

2. Show gratitude by saying thank you. Of course, we all know the polite thing to do is to say thank you when someone opens a doors for us or pays us a compliment, but there are many other things people do that make our life easier in some small way. If you notice the kid bagging your groceries at the store has set aside fragile items like eggs and chips so he can place them on top of other items in your cart, thank him for being so conscientious. When you become a veterinarian, if the receptionist at the front desk schedules some extra time for what she anticipates will be a difficult appointment, notice and

thank her for her thoughtful foresight. If one of your technicians successfully handles a call from tough client, saving you time and energy, even though this may be part of her job responsibilities, acknowledge and thank her for reducing the stress in your day. This is really just a variation of being always on the lookout for good things except in this case you're looking for opportunities to show gratitude to other people.

3. Before falling asleep every night, list three things you're grateful for. These things can be big or small. They can be from the past or present. You can write them down if you wish, but I've found it sufficient to merely think of them while I'm lying in bed waiting to fall asleep. Tonight I'm grateful I get to live in this beautiful place called Flagstaff, I'm grateful I have a wonderful husband who loves me and understands my ongoing battle with emotional reactivity, and I'm grateful I got to watch my dogs run and play in the sun.

PRACTICE #3: Engage in anything that elicits any of the following emotions: Happiness, love, contentment, serenity, curiosity, awe, inspiration, fascination, fulfillment, pride, amusement, hope.

RATIONALE: As mentioned, time spent actively cultivating positive emotions is time spent teaching our amygdala that we're safe. As an added bonus, when you engage in enjoyable activities, you're actually building new skills and learning new ways of thinking. These are long term benefits that can be at your disposal in any situation.

In her 2001 article on the topic of positive emotions, Fredrickson explains that active cultivation of positive emotions over time makes us more creative and flexible, more open to new information and able to integrate that information in innovative ways. This endows us with a broader array of thoughts and actions, a wider variety of possible responses to choose from when faced with adversity.[4] It also makes us more interesting and fun to be around.

As a stereotypical, type-A, overachieving 'gunner,' (which most veterinarians and future veterinarians are) I have always had a hard time allowing myself the space to just have fun, to indulge in hobbies, to spend time doing anything that wasn't directly contributing to the achievement of a serious goal. There was always so much work to do. How could I waste precious time playing? Now that I'm aware of the rationale and the plethora of scientific research demonstrating the importance of doing things for pure enjoyment, I can give myself permission to relax, to savor, to play.

INSTRUCTIONS: No matter how busy your day, find a few minutes to do something enjoyable. Throw a ball for your dog and allow yourself to feel joy as you watch him happily chase it. Spend five minutes watching funny videos on the internet. Find ten minutes to indulge your curiosity about something that fascinates you. And no matter what else is going on in your life, commit to a minimum of one hour (but preferably more) every week to fully engage in an activity that evokes positive emotions for you. Some of the activities I make time for once a week are sewing, reading fiction, planning and cooking elaborate dinners for my husband, and making art.

PRACTICE #4: White Space

RATIONALE: A long time ago, in a galaxy far away, I went to art school. The most precious piece of wisdom I gained from that period in my life came from one of my favorite teachers. She explained to me that in order for a painting to be beautiful, it must have some white space – "places for the eye to rest." In order for our lives to be beautiful, they too must have some white space – a place for our minds to rest.

Do a Google image search for Picasso's *Sleeping Peasants*. The two human figures at the center are surrounded by white space. It's the white space around them that helps us see them more clearly. White space serves the same purpose in our lives: It helps us see everything else more clearly, including ourselves.

If we're in a toxic work environment, or our hospital schedules too many appointments for us to practice good medicine, or we've crammed too many responsibilities into our lives to leave room for any joy - only white space is going to allow us to see those things clearly enough to know we must make a change. The more hectic, busy and chaotic our lives are, the more white space we need. White space gives our subconscious a chance to catch up with us so it can remind us who we really are, so it can tell us what it really thinks about how our lives are going compared to what we'd originally hoped and planned, and what we can do about it.

INSTRUCTIONS: White space is a time when there's nothing to do or accomplish, no one to call, no dishes to wash. It's not for watching TV, or walking the dog, or making to-do lists. It's for nothing. There may be plenty to do, but you're not going to do it, and you're not going to think about it. So there. You're just going to sit here with a nice cup of coffee and look at the clouds.

Or you're going to meander through your yard and look at the trees. Or you're going to sit on your couch and look at the art on your living room walls.

Daydreaming is fine. Being in nature is good. But try to keep your mind unoccupied so you can be receptive to anything your subconscious wants to show you. Make room for a little white space every day, even if all you can do is to pull into a park on your way home from work to stare at the ducks for a few minutes. Try to schedule longer periods of white space every couple of weeks, or once a month, keeping in mind that the more hectic your life is, the more white space you need.

PRACTICE #5: Do Good for Others

RATIONALE: You need to believe you're a good person in order to feel good about yourself. And you need to do good for others on a regular basis in order to believe you're a good person. Veterinary medicine is all about doing good for others. You already know this. But there are many days when a doctor does a lot of good, yet doesn't feel he's done much good at all.

Medicine is complicated. It's rare for a doctor to be certain that what she's recommended or prescribed has a 100% chance of a good outcome. There's a lot of wait and see, and often the answer is ambiguous. When you become a veterinary doctor, do good for others outside the ambiguous arena of medicine, so you can feel good about yourself despite the ambiguity of medicine.

INSTRUCTIONS: Writing a check or making an online donation with a credit card, while it may do good, doesn't give you anywhere near the boost you'll get from doing good in person. So, pick some flowers from your garden and bring a bouquet to work for your hospital's receptionist. Make two quiches for dinner tonight – one for your family, and one that you'll give your neighbor tomorrow morning before you leave for work. If you see an elderly person drop something in the grocery store, rush over and pick it up for him. Go to the dollar store and buy $20 worth of dog treats and spend an hour handing dog cookies out to every dog at the local pound. Send a text to a friend just to say you're thinking of her.

Here's a good idea I heard somewhere: Get a bunch of quart Ziploc bags and fill each one with some moist towelettes, a pack of Kleenex, a travel tube of toothpaste and small toothbrush, some nuts, some chocolates, some mints, lip balm, and a few dollar bills and quarters. Keep these bags in your car. Give them to homeless people you see... Try one of these suggestions or one of your own ideas today, and tell me if it doesn't have an immediate positive impact on how you feel about yourself.

Step 2: Negative Emotional Interpretation

This is the intercept point after which your emotional brain has already made up its mind, so to speak. A decision has been made that something bad or unpleasant has occurred. However, you can still use your thinking brain to stop the negativity cascade from gaining more momentum. You can talk your amygdala off the ledge and prevent it from pulling the trigger on the stress response. You may yet avoid reacting in an emotionally counterproductive way, sparing yourself all of the unpleasant consequences, both internally and externally.

PRACTICE #6: Disbelieve and Dispute

RATIONALE: Disbelieving and disputing unhelpful, negative thoughts is a practice used in cognitive behavioral therapy (CBT). We all have that "inner voice" providing unceasing commentary on everything that happens during every waking moment. Most of us take for granted the validity of what's being said inside our heads. We simply believe it all. But this inner voice does not speak the objective truth.

We can imagine this inner voice as coming directly from the amygdala. It means well. It thinks its job is to protect us and that the best way to do that is by playing the role of a hypervigilant, over-reactive and overly negative backseat driver. Disbelieving and disputing irrationally negative thoughts as they occur, or "cognitive mediation" as described in the 2008 *Handbook of Clinical Psychotherapy,* is an active use of our thinking brain to talk back to the backseat driver in our heads.

INSTRUCTIONS: One of the greatest handicaps I think any of us can have is taking for granted that the voice of that backseat driver is our voice; that it *is* us. No wonder most of us believe everything it says. The more often we question and talk back to (or disbelieve and dispute) the back seat driver in our heads, the more distance we create between the fearful, over reactive part of our brain and our rational, thinking selves - and the wider our stimulus-response space grows.

I've come up with a persona for my backseat driver. Since my tendency when I'm upset is to become angry and combative, I chose the Klingon Lursa. I imagine her with that perpetually angry facial expression (thanks to those Klingon forehead ridges) ranting in Klingon from the backseat of my brain.

This helps me distance myself from the pernicious negativity of my inner voice. It stops me from taking my own irrational anger too seriously and helps me remember that yes, there is some Lursa in me, but I am not Lursa. If your inner voice is more neurotic than angry, perhaps

Woody Allen would be a good persona for your backseat driver. If your inner voice speaks mainly of doom and gloom, maybe imagining Eeyore from Winnie the Pooh would help.

When your practice manager said to you at the end of your very long and difficult first day as a doctor, *"Several of the staff felt you were harsh with them today; apparently they felt you spoke to them in a demeaning way."* What were your initial thoughts? Try putting yourself in an expanded stimulus-response space by distancing yourself from them. Does it help to imagine those initial reactive thoughts as being spoken by the comical persona you've assigned your backseat driver?

Since I've actually been in this situation, I'll give you the PG rated version of what my first thoughts were: *'Who is saying what about me behind my back?! X#$@!'*

After that, my thoughts descended into a kind of pissed off paranoia, where every one of the support staff was suspect in my mind. I was convinced they all 'had it in for me' and that I couldn't trust any of them. It made me feel isolated, bitter and standoffish. And believe me, it added greatly to the stress of being a new doctor.

Now let's try disbelieving and disputing those thoughts – essentially, talking back to them. This is an exercise many do using pen and paper, especially when they first begin practicing it. In time, you can develop the ability to do this in your head so quickly you'll be able to stop a negative knee-jerk reaction in its tracks.

In the left-hand column of the following table, I've expounded upon my initial thoughts (i.e., Lursa's thoughts). In the right-hand column, I've listed alternative interpretations to suggest to Lursa. First, read all of Lursa's negative emotional interpretations, then pause for moment to acknowledge how those statements made you feel. After you've finished with the left column, read everything, top-to-bottom in the right-hand column.

Lursa's negative emotional interpretations	Alternative interpretations to suggest to Lursa
All of the staff are talking about you behind your back. They're stabbing you in the back! Those nasty, petty, little, back-stabbers.	More likely, it was only one or two people and not the entire staff. Secondly, these staff members were probably too intimidated to tell you directly that you had upset them. Doctors are at the top of the power hierarchy in a veterinary hospital, and support staff are typically younger, less experienced and much

	less confident. They probably felt their only option was to talk to the office manager.
They knew your mind was occupied with more important issues, and that you were concentrating on the medicine and worried about a patient. How could they be so selfish? Don't they care that patients' lives are on the line? That your conscience as a doctor is on the line? That your very license could be on the line if something goes wrong? But no, all they care about is making sure they get treated like the precious little special snowflakes they think they are.	The support staff are all here because they care about animals, just like you do. They're just not able to understand the medical situation from your perspective. They have no idea of the thoughts running through your mind, nor of the stress and terror you feel when things are not going well. Remember when you were a veterinary assistant? You had no idea what was really going on, or what the vets were thinking or feeling! If you speak harshly, it's natural for support staff to take it personally. Given that they have no idea of the pressure you're under, can you really label them as selfish? Can you blame them for thinking their own feelings are

	important? Don't we all think our own feelings are important? Even though you didn't mean to, you obviously did hurt someone's feelings, and you should try to find out who, and how, so you can make amends. You also probably need to work on learning to communicate in stressful situations in ways that decrease rather than increase other people's stress.
What is this? High school? You have obviously had the great misfortune of falling into an environment where gossip and cliques control the social climate. You better watch your back and not trust anyone, since they're obviously all a bunch of two-faced, little brats.	This one incident isn't enough to pass judgment on the entire social climate of the hospital. You just started working here. You don't know any of these people, and they don't know you. You're bound to misunderstand each other in the beginning. With some effort and honest communication, understanding will improve.

Can you see how the thoughts in the right-hand column are more conducive to maintaining a healthy state of mind? Can you imagine how these alternative interpretations would lead to a more positive outcome? If I had known about CBT and the practice of disbelieving and disputing the rationality of my negative thoughts before I started practicing, I could have spared myself (and my co-workers) years of emotional fallout.

Notice however, the thoughts in the right-hand column aren't purely positive. CBT isn't about pretending that everything is fine if something bad has genuinely happened, and it's not about turning a negative thought into a positive one. It's reframing, not repressing. It's actively questioning the irrational presumptions and negative pronouncements of the upset backseat driver in our head, and coming up with more reasonable, alternative interpretations. It's about consciously resisting the gravitational pull of the negativity cascade by actively choosing to look at the world in a way that's most likely to foster growth and positive outcomes.

Step 3: Stress Response

Welcome to Negativityville, where nothing good happens, or if it does, we don't notice it. The sirens are blaring and the road to JFK International Airport has been closed. You're on a one-way flight to the frying pan of

Phoenix, Arizona where you will spontaneously combust in a fit of rage (or some other negative emotion).

Your heart rate is elevated, your breathing is altered and your thinking is clouded. There's a part of you that wants to throw something, and there's another part of you that just wants to walk out the door and never come back. In practice, I often experience this when confronting a difficult client or during surgery when things aren't going as smoothly as I'd hoped.

In some ways, by the time you reach this point, it's too late. The physiological changes in your body have already had an effect on your heart and vascular system. Though the effects of a single stress response are often minuscule, they are additive, and if suffered frequently enough, can lead to heart disease and other serious health problems.

Additionally, whatever the situation or event that triggered this negativity cascade, your amygdala has now stored it as a permanent negative emotional memory – it's just one more piece of evidence, as far as your amygdala is concerned, that you live in a dangerous world and it needs to keep a finger on the trigger. But even here, at the end of your rope, you have the power to limit the damage by abbreviating the stress response.

PRACTICE #7: Breathe

RATIONALE: Recall earlier in the chapter when I explained that the autonomic nervous system is involuntary and not under our conscious control? This is true for every autonomic function except one. There is a single function that is shared between the autonomic nervous system and the somatic nervous system, which is the part of the nervous system we do consciously control. That single shared function is breathing.

You could go through your entire life without ever thinking about breathing, yet you would continue to breathe, courtesy of your autonomic nervous system. On the other hand, thanks to your somatic nervous system, you can consciously choose to hold your breath, blow up a balloon or regulate your breathing when you exercise. When you do take conscious control of your breathing, you create a connection to your autonomic nervous system. This connection can be exploited to stop the physiological stress response, to calm your body and restore power to your thinking brain.

In a series of experiments intended to build on other related research regarding the use of breathing techniques to modulate emotions, Pierre Phillipot at the Université de Louvain in Belgium found that specific emotions (namely fear, anger, sadness and joy) have separate and distinct breathing patterns, and not only were those breathing patterns evident when a person was experiencing the specific emotion, but more importantly, those emotions could be induced from a neutral emotional state by mimicking the breathing patterns associated with those specific emotions.[15] This means you can change your emotional state just by changing your breathing pattern.

INSTRUCTIONS: Pay attention to the physical state of your body and the quality of your thinking. Remember the physical sensations you felt while imagining yourself in the story about your first day as a doctor? Do you remember the rush of conflicted and confusing thoughts and emotions you experienced when your body was undergoing the stress response?

Now that you know how to recognize the signs of a stress response, whenever you begin to notice those physiological and psychological changes, remember this: Breathe, and do nothing else. Don't say anything and don't do anything. Don't even think anything except to focus on your breathing. If someone is waiting for you to respond, let them wait. The wait might be good for them too.

The pattern for joy breathing as described by Phillipot is "regular, moderately deep, slow breathing through the nose" with a "relaxed ribcage" and with no tremors or sighs.[15] Do this until you become aware that your body has relaxed and your thoughts have become clearer. Usually, thirty seconds to a minute should be sufficient. Your goal isn't to induce joy by breathing this way when you're upset, but to counter negativity and abridge the physiological stress response. If you can do that, you can climb back up to step 2, the negative emotional interpretation, and use CBT to talk back to your negative backseat driver.

The Mind-Body Connection

It's finally become common knowledge that we have to take care of our bodies in order to enjoy our lives to the fullest. My father, who was born in 1936, grew up, went to college and started his career before the importance of a healthy diet and physical exercise were widely known and accepted. He was overweight, developed diabetes and recently died of complications of diabetes. Aside from the extra decade of life I believe his diabetes stole from him, the quality of all his years was diminished due to suboptimal physical health.

I remember my father as mostly angry and unhappy for much of my childhood. He was a chemical engineer for the Department of Energy, and I don't think he enjoyed his job. His return from work at the end of the day was not something I looked forward to, since it usually preceded an angry tirade that could last for hours. Once, it was because someone had thrown away an apple core with too many molecules of edible fruit left on it.

Another time, it was because the kitchen sponge was dirty and he believed someone must be using it to clean the floor instead of the dishes.

I remember him staying up late into the night, either reading or watching television, then my mother needing to expend great diplomatic effort the following morning to get him to get out of bed so he wouldn't be late for work. Eating seemed to be the only thing that consistently made him happy. In the mornings, the kitchen counter was invariably filled with remnants of pickled pig's feet, rice, crackers, cheese, and the many other things he had eaten in the middle of the night.

Later, when I was much older, I learned from my mother that my father had taken the job with the Department of Energy after losing his previous job. He had lost his previous job after my mother gave birth to my brother, David, who has Down syndrome. Though my father had never shown anything but kindness to my brother, my mother told me that my father had fallen into a deep depression after David was born.

My father was the first born son of a proud Chinese family who traced their bloodline all the way back to Confucius. By not having a son that could carry on that bloodline, my father had failed his family. My sister was born two years later. She was my parent's last try, I presume, for a boy. After that, they likely felt they could not afford or adequately care for more than three children, especially since one of their children had special needs.

While I spent much of my life fearing and resenting my father, in retrospect I understand that he was deeply depressed. His depression led to the sleep disturbances and over eating that negatively affected his physical health, further worsening his depression. After he developed diabetes, he suffered a major stroke that left him paralyzed on one side of his body. Diabetes causes, as one of its major complications, vascular disease, and vascular disease dramatically increases the risk of stroke.

The doctors told me they believed he had likely suffered many previous "micro-strokes" before that, which would have explained the decline in his mental faculties that I started detecting more than two decades before his death. Now that he's gone, I feel only sadness and pity. He did the best he could to provide for our family despite being under what I'm sure must have been tremendous pressure, and he had no other outlet for all of his stress and sorrow.

I can't help but wonder - if my father had taken better care of himself, if he had controlled his weight and taken up jogging or racquetball or swimming when I was young, how differently everything might have turned out. At least, he could have spent the forty-six years of life remaining to him after my brother was born as an active and healthy person. And what would that have looked like? What kind of person would he have been?

I can picture him coming in the door after a jog thorough the neighborhood, wearing maroon shorts and a tank top, dripping with sweat, and raising a muscled arm to dab the sweat away with a towel. That would have been a completely different man. That would have been a man who had taken control of his life and his emotions, and who was determined, despite any sorrow that life might throw his way, to stay healthy and vibrant. Of course, I would expect he'd always have the scar of sadness from never having a son to carry on his name, but if he had transmuted his sadness and rage by redirecting that energy, things could have been different.

Unless you keep your body in great physical condition and already exercise regularly, you may think I'm overestimating the power of diet and exercise, but people who enjoy high levels of physical fitness will tell you, unequivocally, that it has dramatic positive effects on every aspect of their lives. I realize this may not be politically correct right now. Too bad. The truth is a healthy, physically fit you is not going to be the same person as an overweight, out of shape you. Since the focus of this book is to give you realistic expectations about what it's going to be like to be a small animal veterinarian and to provide concrete advice on how to proactively prepare for a long and happy career, I cannot neglect to mention the importance of taking care of your body.

As I've already mentioned, I developed depression within the first year of practice, and it continued and grew progressively worse up to my fourth year of practice. I tried many different anti-depressants that only marginally alleviated my symptoms. Talk therapy helped as a kind of safety valve that allowed me to blow off steam, but it offered no obvious lasting decrease in the depth of my depression. I turned to food as an emotional salve, just as my father had. I'm 5'3" and, at my heaviest, I weighed 184 pounds. That put me soundly into the obese category.

I developed anxiety and had great difficulty falling and staying asleep. The sleep disturbances were exacerbated by working overnights, but persisted even after I transitioned to day practice. I was prone to rage (as my father had been) and ruminations of hopelessness. I started abusing alcohol to dull my anger, and also because the only time I seemed capable of laughing was when I was drunk.

All of this culminated in my therapist reporting me as a suicide risk. Police knocked on my door early one morning and forcibly took me to the ER, where I spent the day on lock-down before being transported against my will to the psychiatric unit of a different hospital. There I spent another 24 hours waiting to be evaluated by the psychiatrist, who finally released me.

While I was in the hospital, blood work was performed and I learned I was pre-diabetic. Something snapped. As awful and terrifying as it was to get thrown into a psych ward, the universe had given me a great gift: Forewarning. Thanks to my diabetic father, I knew what the future would look like if I didn't take proactive and drastic measures to turn my health around. Spending two days in the hospital against my will also gave me a break from my frenetic schedule. I had white space, and the chance to see more clearly the road I was on. My subconscious got to throw a few important questions my way. Was I going to allow this downward spiral to continue? Did I plow through eight, hard years of higher education only to allow myself to become this physical and emotional wreck? Is this the road to the future I wanted for myself? Is this who I wanted to be?

After that incident, I made up my mind to make physical health my number one priority. I bought a treadmill and started using it regularly. I attended a seminar where I learned from an MD who specialized in weight loss that, no matter how much you exercise, if you don't limit your caloric intake, you are not going to lose weight. I started counting calories in addition to exercising. I started losing weight. The more weight I lost, the better I felt and the more motivated I was to keep improving. I started doing power yoga. I lost more weight. I increased my strength and muscle tone. After three years, I'm back in the "normal weight" category.

Although my objective was merely to avoid developing diabetes, and I had no expectation that those efforts would directly improve my emotional wellbeing, regaining my physical health dramatically reduced the symptoms of my depression. It seemed the anti-depressants only started working effectively once I regained my physical health. As the depression started to lift, I found the motivation to investigate and begin meditation and the other practices I recommend in this book, which help me to maintain emotional balance.

While I know being overweight and out of shape didn't cause my depression, I also know, without a doubt, those factors increased my risk for developing depression, and they made my depression refractory to treatment. A 2016 online New York Times article cites a retrospective study published in the journal *Preventative Medicine*. That study analyzed data gathered on more than a million men and women, and found that people with "the lowest fitness were about 75% more likely to have been given diagnoses of depression than the people with the greatest fitness."[48]

Health is a multifaceted gemstone balanced atop a three-legged stool perched on a precipice overlooking a gaping abyss. The legs of this stool are physical well-being, mental well-being and emotional well-being. Compromise any one of these legs and the jewel that makes life worth living, your health, may slip into the abyss. Unlike my father, I was lucky enough to catch this jewel before it fell out of reach. Nonetheless, I had to climb hand over hand back out of that abyss carrying this gemstone between my teeth. It took a long time and great effort.

For veterinarians, being in poor physical condition has more obvious disadvantages as well. When I was an overweight fourth year veterinary student, I had to do a lot of hard physical labor. Carrying all that extra weight made it difficult for me to perform the physical labor required. Additionally, I was awkward and clumsy, and when I lost my balance, or slipped, or tripped, the bulk of my body prevented me from recovering my equilibrium in time to avoid injury. I suffered multiple strains and sprains, and even a permanent injury to my ankle called a talar dome lesion, which still causes me pain, and requires me to wear shoes with a minimum 15mm heel drop.

Successfully completing vet school clinical rotations will not be the end of the physical labor required of you. Many people don't know this but being a veterinarian is a physically demanding job. When my husband was doing his internal medicine residency, he told me about a patient he saw on one of his clinic days. The patient was about eighteen years old but had Down syndrome, and like my brother, was extremely low functioning. He could not speak or express his wishes and he could not be made to understand why he was at the clinic. His mother had brought him simply to have some stitches removed from a laceration repair two weeks prior.

The patient's mother was adamant that sedating her son in order to remove the stitches would take longer and cause more distress than simply restraining him. It took four people to restrain this patient, including my husband, who had to straddle the patient's chest while he removed the stitches. As my husband was complaining about how physically difficult it was for him, I just laughed and said, "Welcome to my world!"

Except in my world, what he described applies to almost every patient, every day. Vets have to help with patient restraint and lifting. For larger dogs, vets need to kneel on the floor to perform physical exams, draw blood and place IV catheters on very strong, sometimes not very nice, and almost invariably uncooperative patients. Vets need to be on their feet, hurrying from exam room to exam room and all over the hospital for long hours, many days out of the week, and they need to stoop over patients for hours as they perform procedures and surgeries. Most procedures require bodily contortions of one variety or another. I have a saying. "Your day as a veterinarian isn't complete until you find yourself suturing upside down in your own shadow."

Think of your favorite superhero: Superman, Wonder Woman, Batman, or Batgirl. If they were overweight, out of shape and physically unhealthy, how effective do you think they'd be at being a superhero? Of course, Superman had the advantage of being an alien with apparently inherently superior physiology. I don't know if he ever needed to work out or not. But Batman was a mere human and he worked very hard at maintaining his physical fitness. Think Christian Bale in *Batman Begins, The Dark Knight and the Dark Knight Rises*.

Veterinarians are superheroes too. Truly. Your future job is going to be using your super powers (your hard won medical knowledge, skills, judgment, and compassion) in a physically demanding job to help animals and their owners. You, and those you serve, will benefit most if you're in good physical condition.

Current guidelines for physical activity advise a total of 150 minutes a week of exercise,[49] although many argue that's still too low. Let's split the difference and say it's at least a good place to start. 150 minutes a week is only 30 minutes per day, five days a week. Half of this time should be spent doing vigorous exercise where you get your heart rate elevated to about 75% of your maximum target heart rate, which can be estimated by subtracting your age from the number 220. For example, 220 minus 48 (my age) is 172. 75% of 172 is 129. Let's round up to 130 for the sake of simplicity. This means when I check my pulse during my workout, I should count about 13 beats in 6 seconds.

6 seconds x 10 increments = 60 seconds = 1 minute
13 beats (in 6 seconds) x 10 increments = 130 bpm

The American Heart Association has more detailed information on target heart rate, as well as some helpful charts. I provide a link at www.realize.vet/book1-resources

I've found my sweet spot for exercise to be 40 minutes of vigorous exercise a day (running on the treadmill maintaining a heart rate of 150-165 bpm) and another 60 minutes a day of power yoga, six to seven days a week. This is what works best for me based on my own experimentation over the course of the last three years. Every day that I complete my exercise regimen, I feel amazing. When I miss a day, I feel sluggish and irritable.

The CDC also recommends at least two sessions a week of some kind of strength training. This is why I do power yoga. It is moderately strenuous in terms of a cardiovascular workout, but it's excellent strength training. Thanks to yoga, I have visible muscle definition again in my legs, arms and abdomen. I memorized my favorite yoga routine, so while I'm doing yoga I can listen to podcasts or audio books.

The NordicTrack treadmill I bought from a Sears Outlet store is one of the best investments I've ever made. I don't have to worry about the weather, and I don't have to drive to a gym and work out alongside a bunch of strangers. I can use my home treadmill any time, day or night. Plus, exercising in the privacy of my own home means I don't have to wear clothes! That cuts down on laundry! I just wear a sports bra, socks and shoes!

Now, I'm going to tell you a secret. Okay, a different secret. Well, maybe it's not so secret. Running on a treadmill is boring. I have to psyche myself up to do it every time. I mitigate the boredom with loud, upbeat exercise mixes. I also have an iPad attached to the dashboard of the treadmill so I can play movies just for some visual stimulation. Believe it or not, I've also found that *increasing* the speed and intensity of my run, paradoxically, often makes it more enjoyable. Creative visualization is another tool I use. I imagine I'm teaching an aerobics class and this girl who picked on me in high school is taking my class. She can't keep up! She's breathing like a barking seal! Ha ha! Hey, whatever works! Our brains are powerful tools and we can use them in any way to motivate ourselves to do what we know we ought to do.

I'll tell you another secret about running. Even though I do it regularly and feel great afterwards, the first couple minutes are still miserable, every time. I just push through. I want you to know this so you don't get tempted to quit your exercising just because the first several minutes (or ten or twelve, on bad days) are unpleasant. The typical progression of one of my runs goes something like this:

Minutes 0-3: My legs are made of lead. I hate this.
Minutes 3-6: Well, maybe this isn't the worst thing ever.
Minutes: 6-12: Actually, this isn't all bad.
Minutes: 12-20: This feels pretty good.
Minutes 20-30: Woohoo! I feel great!
Minutes 30-40: Houston, we have lift off! Yes! I am Wonder Woman! I am invincible! My body is so strong I can practically fly!

We're all different in terms of what combination of types, frequency and duration of exercise will get us feeling our best. The point is, if you haven't already found your own regular routine for keeping in shape, a good place to start is by following the current guidelines. Then experiment until you find the regimen that works best based on your physiology, personality, schedule, and lifestyle.

Maybe spin classes work better than running for you? Maybe you would do better working out at a gym surrounded by people? Maybe doing Crossfit with a friend is what's going to keep you going? Maybe you'd like pole dancing? Personally, I love having the same exercise routine every day because it saves me the time and energy of coming up with new activities, but maybe variety will keep you better motivated. It's all about what works best for you. You, you, you!

Here's another activity to consider. I haven't tried it yet, but if you're a time-pressed pre-vet or vet student, High Intensity Interval Training (HIIT) may be for you. Research has shown that equivalent benefits can come from just 15 minutes of HIIT as running for an hour on a treadmill, and that just two weeks of HIIT can increase your aerobic capacity as much as six to eight weeks of traditional endurance training.[50] A sample fifteen minute HIIT regimen could be as simple as running as fast as you can for one minute, and then walking for two minutes, continuing this sequence for a total of five repetitions. I list several recommended books on HIIT on my website. If you decide to try HIIT and it works for you, shoot me an email and let me know!

If you're not in shape, please, start working on building your physical health now. Anyone seriously thinking about becoming a veterinarian must have a great deal of inner grit. Use that grit to push through any discomfort and mental resistance. I promise if you push through the difficulties of beginning, you will want to scream from the rooftops that it was worth it when you become physically fit.

The hardest part is going to be persevering through the initial unpleasantness. Until your body acclimates to regular exercise, your brain will persistently try talking you out of it. You'll have to push through physical discomfort and psychological resistance for every workout for probably the first several months. But... Just do it!

If you persist, you'll notice subtle improvements that can help motivate you to keep going. You'll notice you feel better when you exercise regularly. Eventually, once you attain a certain level of fitness, it won't be so much about pushing through as it will be about genuinely enjoying your work outs. You'll revel in the feeling of increasing strength and stamina. You'll feel clear headed and optimistically in control of your health and life, rather than foggy, lethargic and irritable.

Perhaps the best thing about being in shape is you'll be more in touch with your own body. This will increase your awareness of the connection between your physical and psychological health. You'll be better able to detect subtle changes in your moods, and if these changes begin to look like a troubling trend, you'll have the clarity to take proactive measures that can prevent a downward spiral. If you're already in shape, I applaud you. I hope you won't let anything derail your commitment to taking care of your body as you face the challenges of undergraduate science prerequisites and veterinary school.

For a link to the video of the yoga routine I memorized, as well as information about the app I use to adjust the tempo of my favorite running music, and the app I use to count calories, visit http://www.realize.vet/book1-resources

Requisite caveat: I'm a veterinary doctor, not a human medical doctor, so I must advise you to consult a human medical doctor before embarking on any weight loss or exercise program, especially if you have underlying health issues.

In Closing

"Happiness is a skill that you develop and a choice
that you make. You choose to be happy and then
you work at it. It's just like building muscles,
it's just like losing weight, it's just like succeeding
at your job, it's just like learning calculus."
- Naval Ravikant, founder of AngelList

I know I'm asking you to do a lot of work. I know
anyone on the path to veterinary school is already
working very hard. But, before you put this book aside
and return to your regular routine with the idea that
perhaps you'll try some of these recommendations later,
consider the metaphysical implications of the second law
of thermodynamics, which I paraphrase as follows:

Any system that does not receive a constant input
of energy will inevitably decay into chaos.

What would happen to a beautiful garden without a
constant input of energy? Or the orderly shelves at the

grocery store? Or your bedroom closet? Everything is a system, and every system requires an ongoing input of energy to maintain optimum order and function – including your mind and your body.

Scientists don't like to speak in absolutes. It makes us very uncomfortable to say that something is "always" or "never" the case. Very little in the known universe is "always" or "never" anything. However, I will make an exception in the case of the importance of self-care. If you want to be a happy and successful veterinarian, to live *with* this calling rather than *up to* or *for* it, proactive measures to care for your emotional, mental and physical health on an ongoing basis are absolutely, *always* going to be essential.

For a list of recommended reading related to the topics in this book, go to http://www.realize.vet/book1-resources

 If you found this book helpful, I'd really appreciate if you would leave a positive review where you purchased it online.

Thank you for giving me the privilege of sharing what I know to enhance your experiences as you make the same journey to become a veterinarian that I made years ago. If you have comments or suggestions for improving any of the books in this series, or if you have additional

questions you would like to see addressed on my blog or on my podcast, please fill out the survey at
www.realize.vet/survey

Here's to your future as a happy and healthy Doctor of Veterinary Medicine.

Kindest regards,
Dr. K
Flagstaff, Arizona, February 2017

Index

1. Boychuk Duchscher, Judy E. "Transition Shock: The Initial Stage of Role Adaptation for Newly Graduated Nurses." *Journal of Advanced Nursing* 2009; 65(5): 1103-1113

2. Desbordes, Gaëlle, et al. "Effects of Mindful-Attention and Compassion Meditation Training on Amygdala Response to Emotional Stimuli in an Ordinary, Non-Meditative State." *Frontiers in Human Neuroscience* November 2012. Vol. 6, Article 292.

3. Fredrickson, Barbara L. *Positivity: Top-Notch Research Reveals the Upward Spiral That Will Change Your Life.* New York: Crown Publishing, 2009.

4. Fredrickson, Barbara L. "The Role of Positive Emotions in Positive Psychology: The Broaden-and-Build Theory." *American Psychologist* March 2001. Vol. 56, No. 3, 218-226. DUP of #10

5. Garland, Eric L., et al. "Upward Spirals of Positive Emotions Counter Downward Spirals of Negativity: Insights from the Broaden-and-Build Theory and Affective Neuroscience on The Treatment of Emotion Dysfunctions and Deficits in Psychopathology." *Clin Psychol Rev.* 2010 November ; 30(7): 849–864.

6. Hersen, Michel, et al., ed. *Handbook of Clinical Psychology; Volume 2 Children and Adolescents*. Hoboken, New Jersey. John Wiley & Sons, Inc. 2008.

7. Hofmann, Stefan G., et al. "Loving-Kindness and Compassion Meditation: Potential for Psychological Interventions." *Clin Psychol Rev.* 2011 November ; 31(7): 1126–1132.

8. http://ei.yale.edu/what-is-gratitude

9. https://en.wikipedia.org/wiki/Amygdala

10. Karlsson, Hasse. www.psychiatrictimes.com "How Psychotherapy Changes the Brain." August 11, 2011.

11. Kearney, David J. et al. "Loving-Kindness Meditation for Posttraumatic Stress Disorder: A Pilot Study." *Journal of Traumatic Stress* August 2013, 26, 426–434

12. Laugharne , Jonathan, et al. "Amygdala Volumetric Change Following Psychotherapy for Posttraumatic Stress Disorder." *The Journal of Neuropsychiatry and Clinical Neurosciences* June 3, 2016.

13. Morin, Amy. www.forbes.com "Developing an 'Attitude of Gratitude' is One of the Simplest Ways to Improve Your Satisfaction with Life."November 23, 2014.

14. Nett, Randall J., et al. "Risk Factors for Suicide, Attitudes Toward Mental Illness, and Practice-Related Stressors Among US Veterinarians." *Journal of the American Veterinary Medical Association* October 15, 2015. Vol. 247, No. 8, 945-955.

15. Philippot, Pierre, et al. "Respiratory Feedback in the Generation of Emotion." Université de Louvain, Louvain-la-Neuve, Belgique and Université du Québec à Montréal, Canada made possible by a grant from the Fonds National de la Recherche Scientifique de Belgique.

16. Shonin, Edo, et al. "Buddhist-Derived Loving-Kindness and Compassion Meditation for the Treatment of Psychopathology: a Systematic Review." *Mindfulness* October 2015, Volume 6, Issue 5, pp 1161–1180

17. Stokes, Timothy B. http://www.amygdalascripts.com "Brain Scans: Five Healing Insights that Advance Psychotherapy and Self Help." March 12, 2013.

18. Tweed, Mike J., et al. "How the Trainee Intern (TI) Year Can Ease the Transition from Undergraduate Education to

Postgraduate Practice."*Journal of the New Zealand Medical Association* 16 July 2010, Vol. 123, No. 1318.

19. Van Dussen, Allison. www.forbes.com "How to Train Like an Olympian." July 8, 2008.(8)

20. Wise, Cari. www.vetprep.com "Vet School, Would You Do it Again? Thoughts on Why So Many are Saying No." June 15, 2016.

21. www.quora.com/Veterinary-Medicine-How-many-veterinarians-are-there-in-the-world

Made in the USA
Monee, IL
14 October 2020

45015265R00075